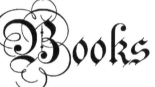
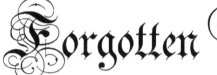

ISBN 978-1-330-28402-5
PIBN 10013019

1 MONTH OF
FREE
READING

at
www.ForgottenBooks.com

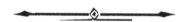

By purchasing this book you are eligible for one month membership to ForgottenBooks.com, giving you unlimited access to our entire collection of over 1,000,000 titles via our web site and mobile apps.

To claim your free month visit:
www.forgottenbooks.com/free13019

A MANUAL

OF

DENTAL MECHANICS

BY

OAKLEY COLES

LICENTIATE IN DENTAL SURGERY OF THE ROYAL COLLEGE OF SURGEONS; DENTAL
SURGEON TO THE NATIONAL DENTAL HOSPITAL, AND TO THE HOSPITAL
FOR DISEASES OF THE THROAT

WITH ONE HUNDRED AND FORTY ILLUSTRATIONS

Second Edition

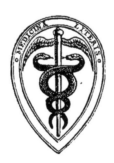

LONDON

J. & A. CHURCHILL, NEW BURLINGTON STREET

TO

ROBERT HEPBURN, Esq.

FIRST LECTURER ON DENTAL MECHANICS AT THE LONDON SCHOOL
DENTAL SURGERY

THIS WORK IS DEDICATED

AS AN

EXPRESSION OF SINCERE RESPECT AND REGARD

BY

THE AUTHOR

PREFACE

SECOND EDITION

In a little more than two years the First Edition of the Manual of Dental Mechanics was exhausted. Sufficient evidence was thus afforded that such a book was needed, and it is not unwarrantable to suppose that the want in some measure was met by the earlier edition of this work. It has been translated into French, and has met with a favorable reception in the United States.

The Second Edition I have endeavoured to make worthy of the consideration with which

its predecessor was received.   Availing myself
of the criticism of my Reviewers, I have endeavoured to so modify and revise this edition
as to bring it down to the present time, and
make it worthier than the first issue of the
recognition of the Dental profession.

5, UPPER WIMPOLE STREET, CAVENDISH SQUARE;
          October, 1876.

PREFACE

THE present work makes no pretence to originality, and is intended for the Student rather than the Practitioner.

Within the bounds of a handbook I have endeavoured to give information of a purely practical nature upon all matters relating to Dental Mechanics, excluding, as far as possible, everything of doubtful value or merely theoretical interest. I may have carried my attempt at brevity to an extreme extent, but noting the present rage for " big books," this is a fault that I trust will be forgiven in a work that is entitled ' A Manual,' and should not, therefore, extend beyond moderate limits.

To the questions of the greatest interest

I have devoted the most space, while many details I have passed over with but brief notice, since they can only be properly acquired in the Dental Laboratory.

I have collected information from many different sources, and have given the knowledge thus obtained, as far as possible, in the words of the original author, so that proper credit may be awarded where it is due. To my American brethren I am under deep obligations for valuable investigations and new facts in the Science of Dentistry.

To Mr S. S. White, of Philadelphia, my thanks are due for the great good nature with which many woodcuts for illustrating the present work have been supplied.

To Messrs Ash and Sons, and Mr G. W. Rutterford, of this city, and Mr Fletcher, of Warrington, I am also indebted for similar courtesies.

I am especially obliged to Mr G. H. Makins for the readiness with which he not only supplied me with illustrations for the section on " Assaying " but also sent notes of the additions to the letter-press that he proposed making to the second edition of his work on 'Metallurgy.'

In conclusion, I may state that this volume has been prepared during spare moments in the course of heavy professional work, and on this account I would ask that it may, in some respects, be leniently judged by my critics and readers; at the same time I trust it will be found useful by those for whom it is especially intended.

O. C.

81, WIMPOLE STREET, CAVENDISH SQUARE
March 25th, 1873.

CONTENTS

SECTION III

THE VARIOUS MODES OF APPLYING HEAT EMPLOYED IN THE DENTAL LABORATORY

SECTION V

PRECIOUS METALS USED IN DENTISTRY

DENTAL MECHANICS

SECTION I

THE PREPARATION OF THE MOUTH FOR ARTIFICIAL TEETH

Preparation of the mouth.—This is a practical point on which depends very often the success or failure of any mechanical appliance introduced into the mouth for the sake of appearance or utility.

The most important thing to bear in mind is this, that the mouth should be in a thoroughly healthy and sound state. If the gums are edentulous they should be firm and insensible to slight irritation, and it is above all things important that there should be a normal condition of the salivary and mucous secretions.

When there are teeth standing they should be carefully examined, any tartar attached to them thoroughly removed, and any carious cavities properly filled.

Any teeth that cannot be restored to a perfectly sound and healthy condition should be extracted, including those that from absorption of their roots, or death of the periosteum, have become loose, although they may not be carious.

Stumps that are quite firm, give no pain on sharp percussion and have no indication of inflammation connected with them around the adjacent tissues, may be cut down level with the gum, and allowed to remain. The pulp cavities however had better be opened up and plugged with gold, or such other material as may be indicated.

If a stump on the other hand is loose, or firm but necrosed or carious, it must be extracted, or, again, if the remains of a broken down tooth are quite firm, give no pain on touching, but slight pain on sharp percussion, and there is a red or purplish tinted line around the gum, then extraction is inevitable. Still, further, if a tooth locally gives no reason for supposing it to be unhealthy, but a gum-boil or scar is discovered near, it will be necessary to remove it.

On all these points no persuasion or assumed direction on the part of the patient must be allowed to influence your own conviction and opinion. Firmness of will is on all accounts desirable under such circumstances. Submission to the wishes of your patient only involves much vexation as a direct result, whilst it defers that which they regard as a great trial until a future time, when the results of the operative interference render the entire readjustment necessary of any artificial appliance that may have been fitted in when the stumps and teeth were intact.

The question how soon after extraction artificial teeth may be inserted, is one of great perplexity if the operator be unguided by practical experience. Theoretically one would conclude that a considerable time should be allowed to elapse, from my own experience, practically I consider twenty-four hours enough, that is, I have many times taken out ten or more teeth one day, and put in a full set of artificial teeth the next day, and I have found the least absorption, especially in comparatively young subjects, in those cases where the shortest time has elapsed between the operation and the insertion of a new denture.

Beyond the advantage of ready treatment which this plan offers, there is the still greater benefit of preserving more completely the contour of the face. Many practitioners consider that a

temporary set of teeth may be fitted in at the
end of a fortnight or three weeks, and a permanent set of teeth at the expiration of twelve or
eighteen months. I have found, however, that
those dentures that I have fitted in immediately
after operating have fulfilled every requirement
of a permanent set, so that no further change
has been necessary.

After removing tartar or extracting teeth,
the following preparation will be found very
useful.

> ℞   Tinct. Krameria, 3j ;
>   Aq. Cologne, 3j ;
>   Aq. Rosæ, ℥viij ;
> As a wash for the mouth; or Potass. Chloratis substituted
>   for the Krameria, according to the condition of the
>   patient.

This may be used as a mouth-wash every two
hours the first day, and thrice daily for a week
afterwards.

SECTION II

ON TAKING IMPRESSIONS

Wax.—For the purpose of taking impressions of the mouth the wax should be pure and well seasoned, if inclined to be brittle and dry it may have a few drops of pure oil added to it while in a melted state and the two well mixed together, this gives a smoother surface and tougher texture than when wax is used alone. It should not contain, however, any spermaceti (with which it is frequently adulterated) or anything likely to reduce its tenacity. For convenience, it may be poured when in a melted state into small earthenware plates, and in this form it is usually sold at the depôts, and can be most readily used.

Softening is best accomplished by immersion in warm but not very hot water; it is better to put the wax into water only luke-warm at first, and then gradually increase the temperature by adding hotter water until the wax is sufficiently soft to be easily moulded in the hand. Each

piece of wax that is intended for use should be
dried thoroughly on a cloth before massing all
the pieces together, this preserves the toughness, and to some extent prevents sucking when
the impression is being removed from the mouth.
The trays for taking the impression, having
been previously fitted to the jaws, should be
kept in the hot water, and when the wax is
ready taken out and thoroughly dried, and even
held for a moment over the flame of a spirit
lamp or Bünsen's burner, this prevents the not
uncommon accident of the tray leaving the wax
in the mouth when its removal is attempted,
as the tray being warmed causes the wax to
adhere firmly to it.

The filling of the tray must depend to some
extent upon the formation of the mouth, but as
a general rule fill up to a level with the free
border of the tray. Keep the impression tray
filled with the wax in the hot water until the
moment you are ready to introduce it into the
mouth, immediately before doing which you
may request the patient to wash the mouth
with cold water. This increases your own
facilities and reduces the discomfort of the
patient. Put one corner of the tray in the
mouth at a time, and thus save painful dis-
tension of the lips, and if it is necessary use

an ivory handled instrument to draw back the angle of the mouth on putting the second corner of the tray into position. When properly in place over the gum to be modelled press the tray firmly and evenly up or down as the case may be. When it is nearly home, with one of the fingers bring all the margins of the wax into close contact with the gums or palate, so that the whole surface of the wax may give a true and not a false impress. In using wax in the mouth I believe too much care cannot be taken in this particular.

When you are satisfied with the position of the tray in the mouth it must be carefully released from the surrounding atmospheric pressure by allowing air to enter under the margins of the wax. This can be done by drawing back the cheeks from along the edges of the impression and also by pushing back the tongue if it be an impression of the lower jaw. The tray should then be elevated or depressed in a line with the direction of the teeth or outline of the gums so as to avoid dragging as much as possible. Cold water may afterwards be poured over the back of the tray so as to harden the wax and prevent the risk of distortion.

Plaster of Paris.—Mistaken notions exist as

to the difficulties attendant on the use of plaster as a material for taking impressions. With a little practice it is quite as easy to manipulate as anything else, and infinitely more certain in its results.

The best plaster only should be used, the water should just have the chill off, and to this must be added (before the plaster) a dram of salt to a quarter of a pint of water.

The plaster must be shaken in so that it does not fall into the water in masses, and when there is enough of it to absorb the water it may be well mixed with a flexible knife, such as a steel palette knife, or better still, an india-rubber paper knife.

The plaster will now be of the consistency of cream, and in this state it may be put into the tray and introduced into the mouth. Ordinary trays of the form shown in Figs. 1 and 2 will answer very well if the surfaces be well roughened.

The great secret of saving your patient any discomfort is to have exactly the right quantity of plaster in the tray to suit the case, and then with a steady hand place it well back in the mouth before you let it touch the teeth. After this bring the free border of the back of the tray into contact with the posterior part of the palate, and then press upwards from behind forwards until the whole of the tray embraces the dental arch. Adopting this plan secures two points, you prevent the plaster running backwards and falling on the base of the tongue so as to produce retching, and, with the patient's head bent forward and the chin depressed, bring the overplus to the front of the mouth where it is visible, and, therefore, more manageable. Another advantage to be gained by adopting this method of taking the impression is this—that the operator runs less risk of leaving air in the space between the surface of the plaster and the vault of the palate. Where sufficient care has not been taken to obtain perfect contact between the plaster and every part of the palate, the impression will have a rough appearance, with irregularly shaped concavities on its surface. With a view to giving a means of escape to the imprisoned air, Mr Turner has suggested inserting a small peg of wood or ivory through the tray and plaster in such a direction that it would reach the vault of the palate, and just before carrying the impression tray quite "home," could be removed so as to allow air to be driven out freely without distorting the surface of the impression. When the plaster that remains in the basin will break with a clean sharp fracture the impression must be removed from the mouth: Air having been let in at the sides by drawing away the cheeks and lips, steady downward pressure must be applied to detach the mould from the teeth and gums.

At this point in the process there must be no hesitation on the part of the operator as every moment the hardness of the plaster is increased, and the difficulty of safe removal becomes greater.

A plaster impression must be left for an hour before it is ready for casting.

Hind's composition.—In those cases in which the upper gum is very hard and firm with some teeth standing, and when in the lower jaw there is much loose, flabby, mucous membrane, then Hind's composition is very useful, and, in the latter cases mentioned, it is a really valuable material.

If the upper gums are thoroughly solid then the required pressure does no harm, and a very good impression can be obtained. When in the lower we have those conditions which I have mentioned, there is a great liability of the impression sucking, that is, the composition remains adherent to some portions of the gum, and thus gives a false mould.

Hind's composition by becoming very hard in

the mouth prevents the possibility of this occurring, and enables the operator to obtain a reliable model; whereas in using wax he would, in all probability, have a false one.

Hind's composition can be softened like wax in boiling water, and the same treatment should be adopted in manipulating it. Stent's preparation was brought out earlier than Hind's, but it requires softening by dry heat to use it to its greatest advantage, the surface also needs coating with grease of some sort when in the tray to get a clean impression, these are objections, besides which, it is wanting in plasticity.

If there are many teeth standing, or a few only in isolated positions, it will require some care lest those materials that possess the property of hardening in the mouth become as troublesome to remove as plaster of Paris.

Gutta percha was largely used a few years back being thought better than wax, and plaster of Paris was not then used to any extent, it cannot however be relied on as it is apt to shrink and it is sticky and troublesome to prepare for use.

Amongst the combinations of the materials I have mentioned, a mixture of wax and paraffin is very good—it toughens the wax, but gives a rather disagreeable smell. Wax and Castor oil will however be found serviceable in some cases ; a dram of castor oil added to a pound of wax will very much increase the toughness of the wax without imparting an objectionable flavour.

Impression cups and trays.—These vary in form, and must be adopted in accordance with the size and shape of the jaws and teeth of which we desire to obtain a model.

To dispose immediately of one sort I may say that, in using plaster of Paris in the upper jaw, only the full-palate tray is reliable. Of these the best forms are those shown below.

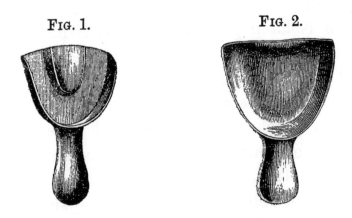

Fig. 1.   Fig. 2.

For wax, Hind's, Stent's, and gutta percha, other forms are available, such as those shown in the annexed engravings, by means of which we take an impression of only a part of the palate and dental arch for the purpose of fitting in a small number of teeth, or it may be an entire upper set, retained not by means of a suction palate plate, but with spiral springs connected with a lower piece or set.

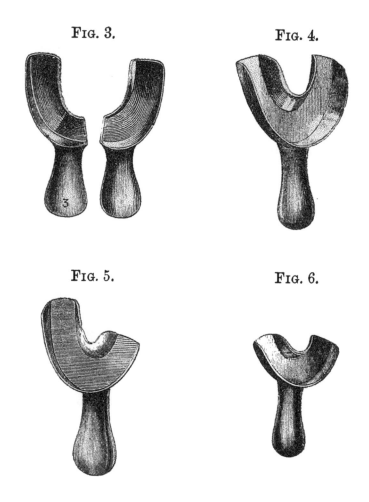

FIG. 3.   FIG. 4.

FIG. 5.   FIG. 6.

When plaster is used in trays it is always necessary to roughen them with a scorper or three-pointed file, and it is very useful to adopt the same plan with the trays used for any of the plastic materials, as it prevents the liability of their leaving the smooth metallic surface.

For the lower jaw it is sometimes requisite to make a special tray, though this but seldom happens; the method of preparing these trays will be described therefore under the head of Special Cases.   If plaster is used for the inferior maxilla, then the best form of tray is that shown in Fig. 7.   A thin strip of 'wax is

FIG. 7.

FIG. 8.

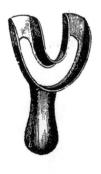
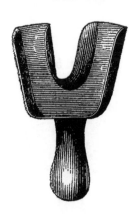

attached to the lower border of the tray, and this is pressed on the surface of the gums, the wax will keep the saliva from flowing into the plaster when it is introduced into the mouth. In taking the impression, I prefer to fill the tray in the mouth when it is in position, pouring the plaster through the opening at the top of the tray, shown in the engraving Fig. 7.

In the lower jaw I have found this a very useful expedient. For the other materials the trays shown below will be most useful, varying the size according to the age and development of the patient's jaws.

Fig. 8.—For cases in which there are teeth remaining at different parts of the jaw.

FIG. 9.   FIG. 10.

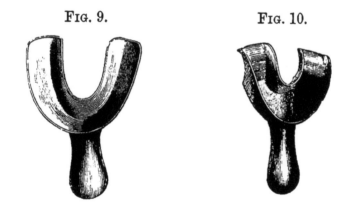

Fig. 9.—For those cases in which the jaw is entirely clear of teeth.

Fig. 10.—For those cases in which the lower front teeth remain, but the bicuspids and molars are lost, beyond this use, the form shown above is advantageous, on account of leaving room for prominent molars in the upper jaw, a condition very often associated with a loss of the lower molars. When from the loss of their antagonists the remaining teeth have become elongated, it is occasionally very difficult to withdraw the impression from the mouth, on account of the small space left between the lower jaw and the upper molars. -

SECTION III

THE VARIOUS MODES OF APPLYING HEAT REQUIRED IN THE DENTAL LABORATORY

The blowpipe.—This is the readiest and most common appliance in use by the dentist for heating a small surface, soldering, and melting gold and its alloys, in quantities up to three or four ounces. The ordinary blowpipe consists of a brass tube about half an inch in diameter at one end, and gradually tapering down to an aperture into which a full-sized sewing-needle can be passed. They vary in length from six to ten inches, and are bent with a sharp curve about one fourth of their length down, so that the fine portion is at right angles to the stem.

If the blowpipe be used for a long time the moisture from the lungs is apt to accumulate and condense in the stem, and become ejected on to the metal being soldered or melted. To provide against this, it is well to have one of the form shown in Fig. 11 with a bulb in the

2

middle of the tube so that any accumulated

FIG. 11.

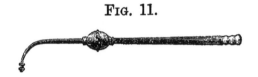

moisture may flow into it and allow of the free passage of dry air.

The danger indicated only happens, however, when the lungs are used for the supply of air. Many prefer a blowpipe that can be used with a bellows, so as to save the exertion and injury that may follow the working with the mouth-blowpipe, in those who are delicate or have any pulmonary affection.

It is impossible to enumerate all the various forms of blowpipe that have been introduced for acting without the aid of the lungs.

The simplest is that shown in the annexed woodcut, Fig. 12, by using which a continuous blast is kept up with but slight pressure of the foot upon the bellows.

The same principle can of course be applied in many different forms. Thus, many prefer to use the Burgess blowpipe, with the bellows arranged underneath, as shown in Fig. 13.

A more important point is the increase of heat and economising of the heating material,

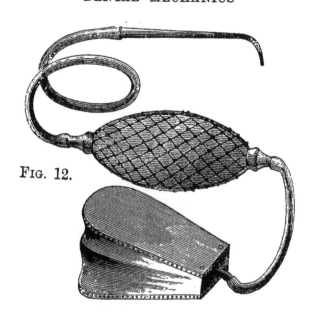

FIG. 12.

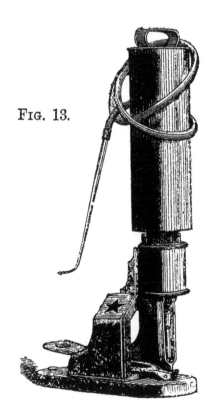

FIG. 13.

whether it be gas or spirit. This, again, has received great attention, and an infinite variety of blowpipes have been invented in order to obtain the best result. One of the simplest, known as "Owen's Blowpipe," is shown in Fig. 14. The gas and air are discharged by two

FIG. 14.

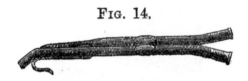

tubes running parallel with each other. Another, invented by Mr. Snow, is seen in Fig. 15, and possesses the advantage of keeping only a small

FIG. 15.

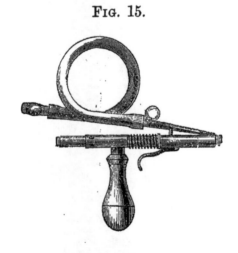

jet of gas alight when hung up by the ring in the upper tube.

A simple form of blowpipe has also been

introduced by Mr Fletcher, of Warrington, in which the tube moves by a swivel in all directions. This can be worked either by bellows or with the mouth.

FIG. 16.

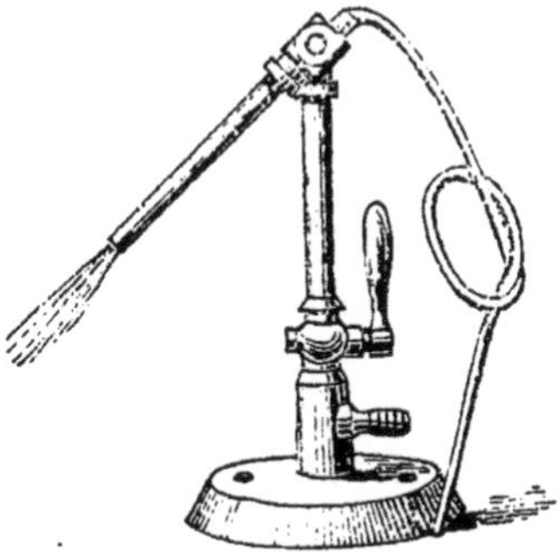

The best blowpipe, however, and one producing the most powerful flame, is that known as

FIG. 17.

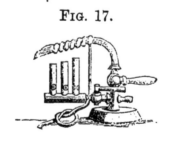

the " Hot Blast Blowpipe," also invented by Mr Fletcher.

The heat produced by this instrument is so great that steel wire burns in the flame, and five or six strands of fine platina are instantly converted into a bead. The intense heat is produced, as will be seen in Fig. 17, by the introduction of Bunsen's burners into the appliance.

Yet another class of blowpipes has to be mentioned, "The Self-acting."

These instruments produce a jet by the evaporation of alcohol, the lamp being so arranged as to convey heat to an upper chamber containing the spirit, which, becoming vaporised, sends out a current with sufficient force to take the place of a mouth or bellows blowpipe.

Three forms of self-acting blowpipes are shown in the accompanying engravings ; one, Fig. 18,

FIG. 18.

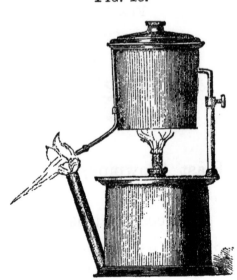

an American invention ; and the other, Fig. 19, of French origin ; while the third pattern is English. In the last-named (Fig. 20) the heat

FIG. 19.

FIG. 20.

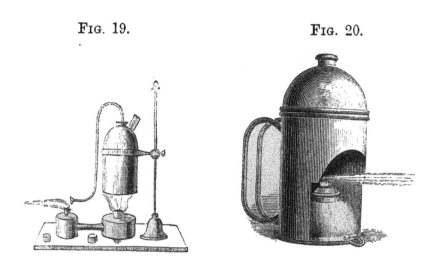

from the lamp below vaporises the spirit in the upper chamber and then ignites it.

Gas is of course the most convenient agent for producing heat in the dental laboratory ; and for using the mouth-blowpipe the best form of burner is seen in Fig. 21. A large volume of flame is obtained from the enlarged end of the pipe, which is packed with layers of iron gauze. This burner is fitted also with a small supply pipe running forward to the end, so that it may constantly have a small jet ready to light the larger burner. When it is impossible to obtain gas, oil or spirit lamps are used. Oil is very objectionable on account of the smoke and the disagreeable smell, and in the absence of gas,

FIG. 21.

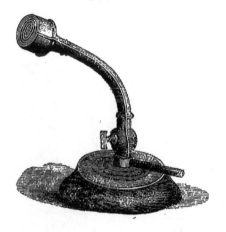

spirit is much more useful. In order to avoid the danger of explosion, however, a somewhat different form of lamp is required to that which is used for oil (Fig. 22).

FIG. 22.

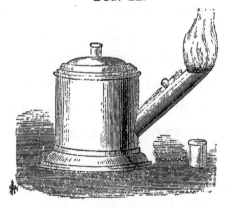

Oil lamp.

A spirit lamp for soldering is shown in Fig. 23. The construction of this lamp prevents the flame being communicated backwards from the wick into the vessel containing the alcohol.

FIG. 23.

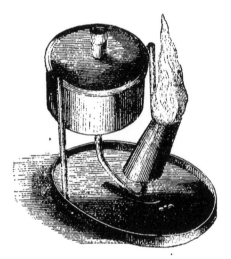

Spirit lamp.

A soldering pan or hand furnace is of great use for the purpose of warming up cases that require soldering, and cooling them down very gradually afterwards.

It consists of a case made of sheet iron, with a grating to hold charcoal, and a cover to keep in the heat; a long shaft with a wooden handle is attached by means of a pivot, which enables the operator to turn it round at will. It is

shown both with and without the cover in the
annexed woodcut, Fig. 24.

FIG. 24.

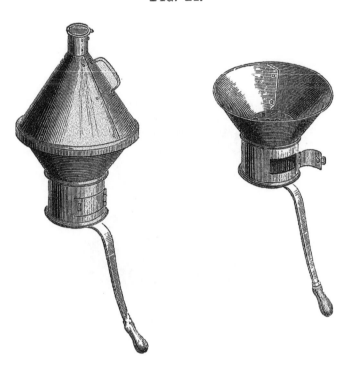

The piece may remain in the pan while it is
being soldered, and so reduce the amount of
heat required by the blowpipe.

Two other modes of applying heat remain to
be noticed, the melting furnace and the furnace
for continuous gum work.

In Fig. 25 is seen a furnace (Ash and Sons')
composed of fire-clay, requiring to be supplied

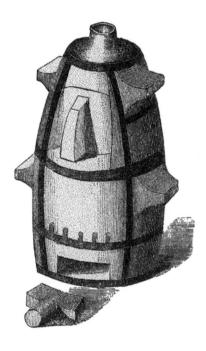

Ash and Sons' furnace for melting gold,
silver, &c.

with charcoal and coke; and in Fig. 26
(Fletcher's) we have a construction of iron in
which the heat is produced by a cluster of
Bunsen's burners arranged within a circle;
both are very powerful,. but Fletcher's being
supplied by gas is the more readily worked.

The furnace for continuous gum work and
gum-blocks is quite different in structure, and
must be supplied with anthracite coal to avoid

Fig. 26.

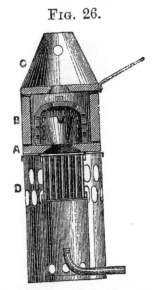

Double-jacket furnace for operating at a white
heat (section).

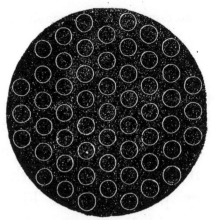

Plan of burner.

any smoke.   A sketch of one is shown in Fig.
27.

FIG. 27.

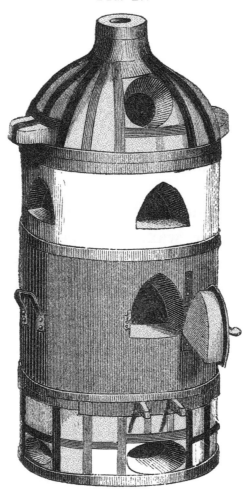

The other varieties of furnaces which are used for melting large quantities of metal are not suitable for use in the dental laboratory. I think therefore it wiser to omit them in a work that is intended to be both practical and concise.

SECTION IV

CASTINGS IN PLASTER AND METAL

To cast a model in plaster from an impression taken in either wax, gutta-percha, Stent's or Hinds' composition :—With all these materials it is wise before casting, to paint over the impression with sweet oil (not thick in consistence) with a camel-hair brush.　A better surface is thus obtained, and the impression more easily separated from the plaster model when cast. If the impression indicates any teeth standing in the mouth in an isolated position they may be strengthened on the plaster model by putting stiff iron wire, pin-size, into the impressions of the teeth, pressing them well into the wax or Hind's as the case may be, to hold them in position while the plaster is being poured.　To avoid the trouble that arises from the oxidation of the wire it is an improvement to use galvanised iron wire or even lead wire such as is used for garden purposes ; or, again, pegs of wood may be inserted; these answer very well for this purpose, dipping them in water before use to prevent the wood swelling during casting.

The shape and height of the model must depend upon whether a gold or vulcanite piece is to be made; if metal castings have to be made then the model in plaster must be high and solid, as seen in the annexed cut (Fig. 28).

Fig. 28.   Fig. 29.

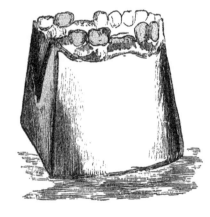

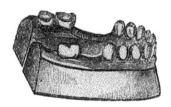

If for vulcanite, however, it may be made very thin and for lower cases of the form indicated in Fig. 29.

Whether the dentures are to be complete or partial the models may be cast according to one or other of these two plans. To prevent the plaster running about and to maintain the desired form a thin strip of sheet lead or zinc, or wax, or gutta percha may be fixed round the impression, the whole resting on a square of paper, so that when the plaster sets the model can be readily removed from the casting bench. The plaster must first be poured into the impression at different points so that it will, with a slight tap of the tray, run down easily into the deeper portions, and when the entire surface is covered with a layer of plaster the eighth of an inch thick, and of the consistence of cream, the portion remaining in the bowl may be thickened and the rest of the model built up. As soon as the plaster is quite hard, the wax can be softened by immersing the impression and model together in a bowl of hot water, allowing it to remain sufficiently long to soften all the impression before attempting its removal. Some prefer dry heat or the flame of a spirit-lamp, from my own experience I think the hot water is the best method, from the fact that there is no liability of the material with which the impression has to be taken melting and sinking into the plaster model.

To cast a plaster model from a plaster impression care must be taken that the plaster impression is quite dry, any mucus hanging about it must be removed by means of boiling water poured over the impression, then with a camel's-hair brush the surface must be painted over with a solution of brown Windsor soap, this prevents the adhesion of the two surfaces of plaster when the model is cast. Dr Richardson ('Mechanical Dentistry,' p. 132) recommends preparing the impression first with varnish to harden it; for this purpose he suggests one or other of the two following formulæ; the first consisting of an uncoloured, and the second of a coloured, varnish;

Transparent Varnish.

Gum sandarach	.	.	.	5 oz.
Alcohol	.	.	.	.	1 quart.

Coloured Varnish.

Gum shellac	.	.	.	.	5 oz.
Alcohol	.	.	.	.	1 quart.

The surface of the plaster having been varnished it is then necessary to coat over this with a thin layer of oil. In my own experience these two coatings reduce the sharpness and fineness of the impression; I would, therefore, recommend the use of a solution of soap. Either plan being adopted the model is made in the same way as if the impression had been taken in wax or some other plastic material. As soon as the model is hard it should be placed in a basin of boiling water and allowed

3

to remain for two or three minutes. The heat produces expansion of the plaster, and the one portion (the impression) having been mixed earlier than the model this expansion is unequal and thus starts the division of the impression from the model, a few taps on the back of the tray will sometimes detach the one part from the other, at any rate it will loosen the tray, and the impression can then be prised off at some point where the greatest loosening appears. Any injury to the model can afterwards be repaired by means of a little plaster. The model is now ready for *trimming up*—that is cutting the sides down evenly, so that they slope slightly outwards, leaving all the surface of the impression untouched within the eighth of an inch of where the denture will extend to. This point is shown and will be best understood by reference to the two last woodcuts.

If the models are to be used for making a vulcanite piece they are now ready; if, however, a gold plate is to be fitted up they had better have the surface hardened by boiling them in a strong solution of alum, borax, melted paraffin, stearine, or a mixture of resin 2 parts, wax 1 part, melted together in a pipkin. Before putting a model into any of these preparations it should be thoroughly dried and then made warm, in this state the plaster absorbs a considerable quantity of any substance in which it may be placed. By one or other of these plans being adopted the plaster is made harder and stronger, and is less likely to suffer from wearing away by the frequent fitting on of a gold plate and bands or collars around the teeth ; it also preserves the prominent markings of the palate and alveolar ridge.

After remaining in the vessel containing the preparation in which it has been dipped for a few minutes, the model must be removed and any superfluous liquid allowed to drain off, and when cold it is ready for use.

Casting in metal.—Casting sand, such as that which is used by brassfounders, should be obtained in a fine state of division and free from dirt or grit. It should be kept in a closed box in order to keep it clear of the dust of the work-room, and made cohesive by adding water four hours before it is used; a little practice will indicate the amount of water required. When ready for use it should form a compact mass if pressed in the hand, and break with a clean fracture. Some recommend using oil instead of water, in that case the proportions are one quart of oil to a peck of sand ; others, again, advise the mixture of glycerine with water to prevent rapid drying, using glycerine one part, water two parts.

The model to be cast must be placed in the centre of an iron ring about four or five inches deep and six or seven inches in diameter; it is well to dust over the surface of the plaster with a little French chalk (soap stone): an ordinary powder puff is the best thing to apply it with. Sand may now be packed all over and around the model and pressed carefully down with the fingers, and filled up to the level of the top of the ring. Now turn it over, run a sharp point round the line of union of the plaster and sand so as to prevent any overhanging portion of the latter remaining, and whilst holding it over the sand box with the model downwards, give two or three taps with a mallet or hammer so as to detach the model and allow it to fall (vertically) into the box; if it is held to one side there is a chance of dragging, as occurs in removing an impression from the mouth in a one-sided fashion.

The mould being ready, the melted metal must be poured in, beginning at the highest and most prominent parts and filling up steadily but not too slowly. Do not have the metal too hot or it will burn the sand and give a rough casting, nor yet too near the setting point or it will give an unsound model. For cases where there are deep undercuts and depressions it will be well to use Dr Hawes' casting ring (Figs. 30 and 31).

FIG. 30.

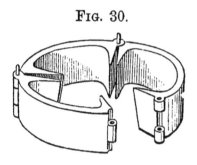

The lower portion, Fig. 30, is divided into three compartments held together with pins, and the upper ring fitted with holes for attachment to the lower part.

FIG. 31.

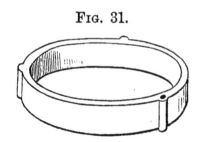

The model to be cast is put into the centre of the lower part of the ring, so that the highest points of the undercuts are on a level with the top of the ring ; it is then surrounded with sand up to the level of the ring, as seen in Fig. 32, leaving the palate exposed. The upper por-

FIG. 32.

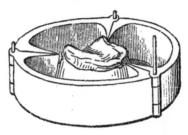

tion of the flask is now adjusted (first dusting over the surface of the sand with French chalk to prevent union) and the whole filled in with sand to the top of the ring. When this is done the upper complete ring may be taken off, and removing one of the pins from the lower ring the sections can be opened and the model removed afterwards ; the whole being closed up again is turned over the reverse way and metal poured in as with an ordinary mould. With lower models, when undercut at the angles of the jaw and at the back of the overhanging front teeth, it is best to fill in first with wax and then trim away with a scorper after casting and while the metal is still soft.

If, however, the undercut is so great that "trimming" up is likely to give an imperfect model, it will be better to adopt the plan that

is in use at the large metal foundries. This
consists of making a mixture of asbestos,
sand, and plaster, and filling in the undercuts
in such a way that the model will " draw." The
model should be dried and dipped before the
" core," as it is called, is cast, and after it has
remained in place sufficiently long to become
quite hard it must be removed and made perfectly dry. It will be readily understood that
cores may be so cast that they will enable the
model to "draw" easily out of the sand in one
direction, whilst from the nature of the undercut, the core itself can only be removed in
some other direction, so it is that we are enabled
to fit the cores in place on the model, obtain a
mould in sand, removing the model and cores
together, and then taking the cores from the
undercuts replace them in the sand, in such a
way that the mould thus completed represents
the whole of the plaster model in reverse.

Still another method of casting dies and
counter dies is proposed by Dr Franklin in Dr
Richardson's 'Mechanical Dentistry,' consisting
of the following process :

" I take all impressions, full and partial, in
plaster. A small hole, less than $\frac{1}{16}$ inch, is
drilled through the highest point of the palatal
surface of the impression, through cup and all;

into this place two or three broom splints
cutting them off even with the surface of the
plaster, to allow any vapours to pass off. I
sometimes smoke the surface of the impression.
Around the impression place sufficient putty to
form a ring the size and height required for the
die. Into this pour, at as low heat as consistent
with the mobility required for sharp castings,
the bismuth alloy known as Sir Isaac Newton
metal, or, which is better in some respects, 8
parts bismuth and 4 parts each of tin and lead
—the latter composition being a little harder.
If a little judgment is exercised in pouring
either of the above alloys, a perfect die will be
secured from moist plaster impressions without
any drying. As the bismuth is expansive, and
the alloy is hard and somewhat brittle, I run
only a thin casting, not more than half an inch
in thickness, over the highest portion of the
impression. I have cast iron or brass heads
made three inches and a quarter in length, three
inches in diameter at large end, and two inches
at the other; the large end is flat and well
coated with common tinman's solder. This
head is heated until the solder begins to soften;
it is then placed in a pan or other convenient
vessel, and the die, face side up, is placed upon
the tinned surface. When the die begins to

melt, and perfect union is secured, cold water is dashed upon the die and head; and thus we have a sharp die, with an iron head, to sustain the force of the blow in stamping the plate, and by this means preventing any spreading of the face of the die or liability of breaking in the process of swaging.

"I now take sheet lead of the thickness of about No. 24 standard gauge, and adapt it to the face of the die by means of a wooden mallet or burnisher, or other convenient means. Trim the lead plate to the size required for the plate to be stamped; when the lead plate is nicely fitted, remove it carefully from the die, and place it in a ring or narrow moulding flask, the palatal side up; now gently stamp moulding sand into the plate and flask up level with the edges of the flask; then reverse the flask and cut the sand away *clean* for half an inch or more down to the edge of the lead plate all around. Around the plate place a common moulding ring sufficiently large to form the counter, which is made by pouring melted tin or lead (or any alloys of these metals) on to the lead plate, being careful not to run the metal so hot as to melt the lead plate. When the counter is cool enough to handle, the adhering sand is brushed or washed away; the die is then placed into the bed or counter, and, with a moderate-sized hammer, give one or two sharp blows to bring the die and counter together. In swaging gold plates, two or three or more dies may be required; these may be made either by running the die-metal into the impression (if not broken), or by running into lead plates, gotten up as before described, reserving, of course, the first die and counter for the final swaging of the plate. I have gotten up a die and counter from the impression, with the aid of an assistant, in the foregoing manner in twelve minutes. I usually get out my die immediately after taking the impression; adapt a wax or gutta-percha plate to the die, and get the articulation before the patient leaves the office."

We have now the *metallic die*. The next step is the counter die. This may be obtained in three ways.

The simplest plan and that most commonly practised is to melt a ladleful of lead, and when the metal is beginning to set dip the model into it, letting it go down a depth sufficient to cover all those parts that the plate is to be fitted to. On cooling, the model can be easily detached by a few blows of the hammer.

Another plan is to place the model on the

casting board, bank it round with moist casting sand, and then put an iron ring on the sand to prevent the lead, when poured over the surface, from running about (Fig. 33).

FIG. 33.

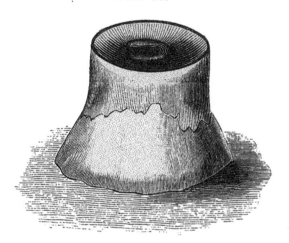

This admits of the greatest pressure falling on the parts where it is most required, and for partial cases is very useful. Or, again, a third mode is to dip from the plaster model. First having provided a shallow iron tray, three or four inches deep and five inches square, pour lead into it, and just as it is beginning to set dip the plaster model in the same way that you would the metallic one; remove the model when the lead is set, and wash away all particles of plaster. For this plan several models must be on hand, as one or two will be destroyed, and before using them be careful that they are thoroughly dry. We may, if we desire, cast the model from this *dip* by putting an iron ring round, driven slightly into the lead, and then pouring zinc into the ring. This last plan, however, is not so good as the ordinary method of casting the zinc model in sand first of all, from the plaster one.

The materials for metallic castings are zinc for the models or dies, and lead for the counter dies. With Fletcher's gas furnace they can both be very readily melted, and answer better than any other metals that can be prepared in an ordinary workroom; there are, however, sometimes occasions on which a more fusible metal than either of these is of great service.

Of these the following are the most useful :*

Type-metal.—Lead 5 parts, antimony 1 part; fuses at 500°.

Zinc 4 parts, tin 1 part; melts at a lower temperature than zinc; contracts less, but is not so hard as zinc.

Tin 5 parts, antimony 1 part; melts at a lower temperature than either of the previosly mentioned alloys, but is easily oxidized; it must therefore be poured quickly.

The following table of alloys, fusing at a still

* Richardson's ' Mechanical Dentistry.'

lower temperature, is given by Professor Austen in the 'American Journal of Dental Science' (vol. vi),

	Melting point.	Contractility.	Hardness.	Brittleness.
1. Zinc	770°	·01366	·018	5
2. Lead 2, tin 1 . . .	440°	·00633	·050	3
3. Lead 1, tin 2 . . .	340°	·00500	·040	3
4. Lead 2, tin 3, antimony 1 .	420°	·00433	·026	7
5. Lead 5, tin 6, antimony 1 .	320°	·00566	·035	6
6. Lead 5, tin 6, antimony 1, bismuth 3	300°	·00266	·030	9
7. Lead 1, tin 1, bismuth 1 .	250°	·00066	·042	7
8. Lead 5, tin 3, bismuth 8 .	200°	·00200	·045	8
9. Lead 2, tin 1, bismuth 3 .	200°	·00133	·048	7

The zinc die and lead counter die will become very hard in striking up the plates; they must, therefore, to make them wear well, be annealed occasionally; this can be done best by putting them together and placing in a ladle with a little water over them; when the water has boiled away allow them to remain for a minute or two longer according to the state of the fire and then cool them down, when they will again work well.

SECTION V

PRECIOUS METALS USED IN DENTISTRY

Gold. (Au.)—*Equivalent* 196·6; *specific gravity* 19·34; *fusing point* 2016°·

Properties.—Extreme malleability, ductility, and tenacity; non-liability to oxidation, and resistance to the action of the simple acids. It is, however, soluble in nitro-muriatic (*Aqua regia*) and nitro-fluoric acids.

Gold, alloyed with other metals, is used in mechanical dentistry in the form of plate, wire, and foil. All of these may be obtained ready for use, of the required thickness and sizes, at our dental depôts; and many dentists with a view of saving the trouble and expense of melting and flatting for themselves, always purchase their precious metals in this way.

Some, however, may not be able to do this on account of location in the provinces or colonies; it will be well, therefore, to give some of the characteristics of gold and particulars of the method of working it into the forms required by dental surgeons.

Gold in the pure state is too soft for use, readily losing its form on comparatively slight pressure; it must therefore be combined with certain other metals to give it the requisite amount of hardness.

Alloys of Gold.—With copper a reddish alloy is formed, very much harder than either metal separately. The copper must be quite free however, from antimony, arsenic, and lead, or a brittle alloy will be the result. The greatest degree of hardness is obtained by combining seven parts of gold with one of copper.

The best alloy for hard wear however (such as coinage), is equal parts of copper and silver, regulated according to the quantity of gold plate or wire required. American gold coins are chiefly prepared with copper only, hence their extreme hardness and red tint.

One other alloy is of interest in this department, that is, a combination of gold, silver, copper, and platinum. This alloy is extremely useful for clasps, bands, pin wire, and other purposes where great toughness and strength are required. The exact proportion of the various alloys useful to the practitioner will be found under a separate heading. Before passing

on to the purely practical part of the preparation of gold for use in the workroom, it
may be convenient to describe a process which,
although of too complex and scientific a nature
to be very well carried out in the dental
laboratory in the midst of the ordinary work of
every day practice, is nevertheless of great
importance; I shall therefore introduce a section on assaying from the valuable Manual of
'Metallurgy,' by Mr Makins.

Assay of Gold Alloys.—"In earlier days of
these operations, when, for commercial purposes, they were not carried to the nicety of
the present time, it was common to make a
kind of rough assay by means of the touchstone, and, in experienced hands, with pretty
good results. The requisites for the process
were a few needle-shaped pieces of gold, of
various known qualities, a piece of a roughish
black stone, and a little nitric acid, of about
1·20 specific gravity. The sample to be
examined had some angular part of it drawn
across the surface of the stone; but, as in
articles of jewellery, the surface is often what
is termed "coloured," and consequently richer,
a few rubs were given of the part to be examined
upon some rough surface, previous to making
this testing line upon the touchstone. The

assayer then took one or two needles which
he supposed to be near in quality to the one
sought.   These are drawn across the stone, and
then the streaks are moistened with the nitric
acid.   If the qualities are nearly the same, the
action of the acid will be nearly similar; if not,
the streak made by the coarser of the two will
be most acted upon, and his experience would
then point out, by peculiarities in the test streak,
which needle he should have to choose for final
comparison, if it had not already been employed
where more than one was first used.   The
practice is, however, a very rude one, and at
best depends too much upon judgment.

"The outline of the operation for the actual
assay of gold is as follows:—An assay pound of
the alloy is first very accurately weighed; next,
pure silver, to the amount of from two to three
times the supposed weight of gold is added;
then this is cupelled with a proper proportion
of pure lead.   The button so obtained is now
flattened somewhat by the hammer, and then
rolled into a ribbon.   This ribbon is annealed
and coiled, and is then ready for the parting
operation, which consists in boiling it twice in
nitric acid, and, between and after the boilings,
washing in water.   Lastly, annealing the gold,
and weighing.   Gold (in assaying operations) is

best weighed decimally. Thus, in a pound, or 1000 parts of English standard gold, we should find 916·66 of fine. The decimal weights may be converted into trade by calculation.

"But the system of trade weights for gold are not the pound divided into ounces and penny-weights, as for silver, but the pound is said to contain 24 carats, each carat 4 carat grains, and these latter are divided into halves, quarters, and eighths; the eighth, or 768th part, being the lowest amount reported. The actual weight of the pound varies much, thus some assayers (those who follow the French directions) use only 7·5 grains, while, on the other hand, English assayers will use from 10 up to 16 grains. The capability of using a tolerably large weight of course assists in the greater delicacy of the small weighings. By a trade report, as it is termed, standard gold, which contains 11 of gold to 1 of alloy, would be said to be 22 carat gold, any specimen containing more would be called "better," and less than that amount " worse." As this method of weighing is still used by many assayers, an illustration or two may be given. Having at first "weighed in" an assay pound of metal, and carried it through the various stages of the operation, the fine piece of gold resulting is placed in the balance;

in the other pan is put the 22 carat, or standard weight. Suppose the gold does not counterpoise this, sufficient weights are added upon the gold pan, and thus, supposing a carat grain, a half, and an eighth, were found necessary, the gold would be reported, W, 0 carat, $1\frac{3}{8}$ gr. If, on the other hand, it was heavier than standard, and weights (say) of 1 carat, $2\frac{3}{8}$ gr. were required to be added to the weight pan, the report would then be, B, 1 carat, $2\frac{3}{8}$ gr. Thus gold of 18 carats fine would be written, W, 4 carats.

"The rough weights of metal for the gold assays being prepared by an assistant, are weighed in for the furnace by the assayer himself, who, judging quality from external appearances, &c., adds to them at the same time the requisite amount of pure (or 'water') silver, and then wraps silver and gold together in a piece of sheet lead, weighing half the amount of the lead required.

"The quantity of lead to be employed will be about 6 times the weight for gold down to about 920. Below that and down to 750, 8 times will suffice. And for qualities below the latter, 10 will often be required, although these proportions are often modified by the presumed nature of the alloy.

"The furnace being prepared and heated just

as described for silver, the assays are charged
in when the heat is judged to be sufficient, and
the cupel operation is then carried on, as with
silver. But the care requisite here is very
much less than in the latter class of assays, the
object being as much the alloying of gold and
silver as the complete separation of oxidisable
metals; because any small amount of the latter
left in the assay will be removed by the acid in
the parting operation, which retained alloy in a
silver assay, where there is no after-assisting
operation, would be just so much of error. A
certain amount of care is, however, to be
exercised for several other reasons; thus, for
example, if assays, and especially gold ones, be
charged into cupels insufficiently 'seasoned'
in the furnace, 'spirting' is sure to result:
this is the throwing up from the bath of fused
metal of a number of small beads of the assay;
these will be projected even to the crown of the
muffle, and falling all around, spoil the assays
in the surrounding cupels.

"Again, loss may accrue from vegetation or
springing if the assays have been carelessly
cooled down; and, lastly, a muffle not properly
cleared, or having a fragment of coal shut up in
it, will, by containing an atmosphere of carbonic
acid, cause reduction of the oxide of lead at the

external parts of the cupel, which reduced lead, being taken by the yet fluid button, will render it so brittle as to fly to pieces under the hammer.

"The flattening hammer requires some dexterity in its use. The buttons being taken from the furnace are one by one placed upon an anvil and struck three blows; the first, a downright one, gives the piece the diameter equal to the width required of the ribbon. The next blow is a kind of drawing one upon the edge, whereby a kind of tongue is drawn out sufficiently thin to cause it to be readily seized and drawn in between the rollers of the flatting-mill. The other end of the assay is then turned round, and a similar blow and conformation given to it.

"The board containing the flattened buttons is now taken to the rolling-mill, and all are passed through, with the rollers set just at such distance apart as will equalise the assays. They are next adjusted down to the distance, which shall elongate the assay into a ribbon of metal required ; and now if the flattening operation with the hammer has been well performed, they should all be of equal breadth, and for an assay pound of 10 grains, measuring about ·4 of an inch wide, the rolling operation, bringing them to 2·2 inches long.

" This treatment of the metal will, however, have rendered it very hard and dense, therefore annealing is required before the parting operation, for which purpose the assays are placed in a solidly made iron tray, each one in a separate division. The tray is put into the muffle and heated to dull redness, after which it is taken out and the ribbons of metal coiled up into small cylindrical rolls, called ' cornets.'

" The requisite number of assay glasses are then charged with from 2 to 3 ounces of nitric acid of a specific gravity of from 1·16 to 1·25 ; and these are arranged upon a gas parting apparatus. This consists of a tube, A, connected with the gas supply, from the upper part of this rises a number of cocks ; and on the outer screw of each of these a cup-shaped burner, B, is screwed, the jets of the burner, passing out horizontally from its circumference, cause the flame from each to wrap itself round the end of the glass. For a small set of from six to twelve burners the arrangement shown in the drawing may be adopted where the whole are fixed in a mahogany stand. This latter is furnished with a set of long tubes, D, one for each glass, C ; and when the evolution of acid vapours commences, they may be inserted in the necks of the glasses, thus condensation of the acid takes

FIG. 34.

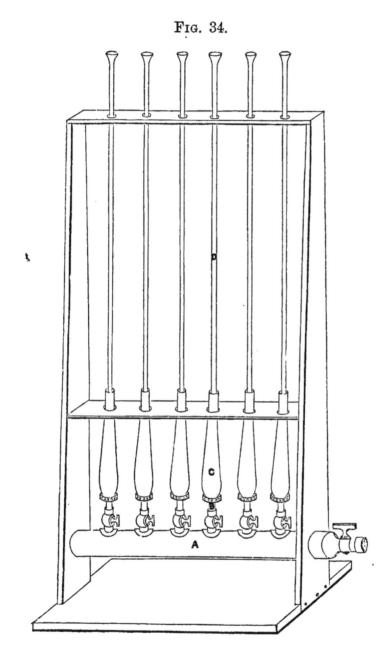

place in them, and the condensed product runs
back into the glass, while the escape of noxious

vapour is to some extent moderated. In an active laboratory, where fifty or more are worked at a time, it is necessary to arrange the whole in some convenient chamber, provided with a flue for carrying the acid vapours away. The tubes D are then dispensed with, and the burners are better to be placed upon two or even three gas tubes, so as to be more under the eye.

"After the assay glasses have cleared of red fumes, from three to five minutes' brisk boiling is kept up, they are then removed from the burners, and the solution of nitrate of silver poured off, the cornets washed with a little hot distilled water, and a fresh dose of acid put into each glass (of a specific gravity of 1·3). They are then boiled again for fifteen or twenty minutes, after which the acid is poured off and the glasses quite filled with warm distilled water.

"It will be found that acid of the above density is apt to boil unsteadily, and its vapours, by adhesion to the sides of the glass, will be given off irregularly and with such violence as even to project nearly the whole of the acid from the glass. Hence it is found necessary to put some body in with the assay, which, by affording points for the evolution of the vapours, shall facilitate its steady delivery from the fluid. For

this purpose the practice by many is to use a
piece of charcoal, but this is apt to induce the
evolution of nitrous acid, which by absorption
in the acid will even dissolve portions of the
metal. This has been proved by the author,
and put forward in a paper lately published
by him ('Quarterly Journal of the Chemical
Society,' 1860). Moreover the acid becomes
much discoloured by charcoal, hence Mr Field,
the Queen's Assay Master, has proposed
the use of small balls of porous earthenware, and these answer the purpose most
admirably.

"The assays are next turned into small
porous earthenware crucibles for annealing, but
the cornets, with the silver now removed, occupy
the same bulk as before parting; hence from
their spongy, and consequent friable nature,
much care is required in effecting this, or they
are sure to break up. The pot is therefore first
filled with water, and the neck of the glass
stopped by the forefinger, then being dex-
terously inverted under the water of the pot,
the finger is removed, and the assay allowed to
fall steadily into the pot, time also being given
for any pieces (if any should by chance have
become detached) to fall on to the assay. In
this operation, if the piece even touch the finger

in its transfer portions are very likely to be detached.

"The pots are now arranged in the furnace, and heated up to an annealing heat, thus the former bulky cornet is condensed and shrunk considerably, while its surface, by incipient fusion, becomes perfectly metallic, changed from the brown lustreless appearance it had when washed off to a pure golden surface.

"It now only remains to weigh the assay, but compensation must be made for a certain retention of silver; this not only varies with different operators, ranging from one to ten grains in the troy pound, but is subject to slight difference with the same assayer, dependent upon the furnace heat, atmospheric influence upon the boiling of the acids, and other disturbing actions. Beyond this there will be, on the other hand, an allowance to be given from the precious deduction for loss of gold during the operation, which is subject to like variation with the silver retention. This averages about one to six grains in the pound troy. Hence the operation can only be carried on to perfection by those who are continually practising it; and in such hands it needs daily tests to be passed with the working assays, as proofs or standards, whereupon to base the necessary corrections to be applied.

" In addition to the operation of assaying for the amount of silver or gold as already detailed, there are cases where it is required to estimate silver contained in gold, and also gold in silver, such are called ' parting assays.' The latter, viz. that of silver contained in gold, is effected by simply dissolving the metal in dilute nitric acid, and collecting the gold powder left ; this is then to be washed with boiling distilled water, and annealed to brightness, when it will be in a state for weighing.

" The valuing of silver in gold is somewhat more complex. A double gold assay is made in the usual way, and at the same time an assay pound of the metal is cupelled with no silver added. Thus the copper and oxidisable metals are removed, and the button left will be composed of the gold and silver of the specimen only. The difference of weight of this above the parted assay will of course be due to silver. But in this operation, not only are comparative assays necessary, but much judgment and experience upon the part of the assayer, or the results will be quite unworthy of confidence.

" In the dental laboratory, where it is pro- bably of advantage to be able to obtain assays upon very small quantities of metal, very good approximate ones may be obtained by means of the blowpipe, with the additional advantage of rapidity of execution dependent upon their smallness. Thus a common candle urged by the blast of the ordinary mouth blowpipe will afford the requisite heat in the hands of a practised blowpipe manipulator ; but where the gas blowpipe, joined with the double bellows already described can be obtained, the operation becomes very easy and certain.

" A grain of gold will be sufficient for the assay pound ; and if to this we add the two to three grains of silver requisite, and seven grains of lead, the whole mass of metal will at first only weigh ten grains, or a little more, according to the amount of silver used, a quantity managed with ease.

" For this a small cupel of about a quarter of an inch each way may be employed. This may be rested in a small cavity cut in a piece of sound charcoal. The tip of the flame is first to be directed on this so as to heat it up somewhat ; after which the assay, prepared as in ordinary assays, is to be put in, and when fused by the flame directed upon it, the cupel is to be kept just in that position in the oxidating flame as will carry oxidation on, and at the same time maintain the heat of the cupel so that the lead oxide may be absorbed ; although much in this operation passes off in vapour. These actions are to be steadily maintained until the assay brightens. It is then removed from the cupel, flatted and rolled. The ribbon may then be annealed by a spirit-lamp, after which it is rolled up, and parted with two acids. These last operations may even be effected in a test tube over a spirit-lamp. The little cornet is, lastly, to be washed into a small porcelain or platinum basin, and annealed over the lamp, when it will be in a state for weighing. And if this operation be well and carefully carried out, very close approximations may be obtained.

" As a most delicate balance would be required for these minute weighings, and such an one is not always at hand, I may state that the little instrument described by Mr Faraday in his ' Chemical Manipulation,' as Dr Black's substitute for a delicate balance, will answer very well for these weighings.

FIG. 35.

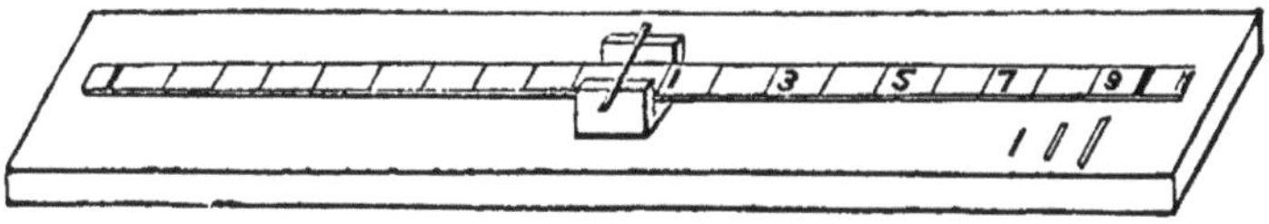

" It consists of a thin slip of pine about twelve

inches long and ·3 of an inch broad in the
centre, but slightly tapering both in breadth
and thickness to each end; in the middle of this
a very fine needle is fixed at right angles upon
its flat and upper side.   Upon each side of this
needle or fulcrum, ten divisions are marked at
exactly equal distances from each other, starting
on each side from the needle.   The bearing upon
which the beam is to play is a small piece of
sheet brass turned up to equal heights, so that
a very narrow plane is thus formed on each side
of the beam for the needle fulcrum to rest upon;
and as this rises only a quarter of an inch from
the little slip of mahogany upon which it is
screwed, the play of the beam is very small.
The beam of course after thus being shaped is
to be adjusted so as to equipose upon this
bearing.

"The weights requisite for decimal weighing
will be three only, viz. one grain (as an assay
pound) ·1 of a grain, and ·01 of a grain; and
these are best formed in platina wire of fit
degrees of fineness, as shown in the drawing,
where they are represented as lying upon the
mahogany base.

"An example may be given to illustrate the
method of using this little apparatus.

"Placing the grain or assay pound weight

upon the 10th or principal division on one end, a slip of the metal to be assayed is cut off, and if of somewhat the shape of the pound, it will be better for accuracy of weighing, as it will lie better upon the beam division, care also having been taken that it should be rather plus, it is to be reduced to the correct weight. Then after cupelling, and parting this as above, the cornet obtained is to be placed upon the 10th as before, and now being diminished in weight by the loss of its alloy, the pound must be passed back upon the beam divisions, but even at one back, or division 9, the weight being found too light for the cornet, it is allowed to remain at 9, and the 2nd or ·1 weight is placed on 8, and being found too heavy is passed back, trying a division at a time, until, arriving at division 1, it is found too little. Hence, leaving the 2nd also, upon division 1, the 3rd or ·01 weight is used in the same manner, and passing it back by divisions its real position would be found to be between divisions 6 and 7. Hence, the weight ascertained is thus reckoned. First, the 1000 or pound weight being upon 9 gives the first figure of the report, viz. 9. Secondly, the tenth of the thousand on the first division gives 1 as the second figure. Thirdly, the hundredth of the pound, requiring to be placed at a point between 6 and 7 may be called 6·5. Therefore the weight will actually be 916·5, indicating the specimen to have been one of standard gold.

" It will readily be seen that if necessary this simple instrument might be equally easily applied to trade weighings, by dividing the beam into 8, as the ⅛th of a carat grain is the smallest denomination, instead of 10 divisions, and then using the 1 grain pound as 24 carats with proportional weights of 22 carats, 2 carats, 1 carat and 1 carat grain. But the decimal method is very simple and its weights are easily convertible."

Melting.—The quality of the gold plate or wire having been decided upon, and the proper relative proportions weighed out carefully, they are to be put into a crucible, varying in size according to the quantity to be melted, always having the crucible a good size in comparison with the " melt," and the metal covered with borax, some of which is also mixed in with it. The pot must be placed in the furnace, with small pieces of charcoal put into the crucible above the borax, and the whole well surrounded with fuel.

The form of crucible best suited for small quantities of metal is shown in Fig. 36.

When the gold is melted and thoroughly in-

FIG. 36.

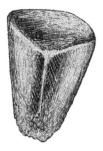

corporated with its alloys, it must be poured
into an ingot mould held in a frame (shown in
Fig. 37). Previous to pouring, however, the

FIG. 37.

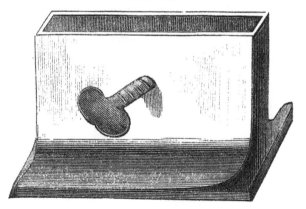

two portions, of which the mould is formed,
must be warmed with a lamp or over the fire, and
then wiped with an oily cloth such as is always
found in use in connection with the flatting mills
and other machinery. This causes the metal to
flow better.

Everything being ready the gold is poured

into the ingot mould, and after a moment or
two being allowed for setting, it is taken out
and dipped in weak acid and water to cool it
and cleanse the surface. Any sharp edges of
metal that are likely to break off had better be
removed at once with the file; it may then be

FIG. 38.

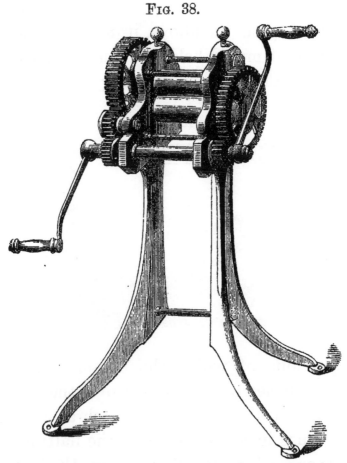

FLATTING MILL on iron stand to fasten to the floor,
with hardened rollers 4 inches long and 2¼ inches
diameter, with a double set of cog-wheels for multi-
plying the power, and two handles (Fig. 38).

annealed by placing on the ashes in the furnace or forge. Some proceed now to flatten the ingot at once in the mills; it is, however, better to forge first, and reduce the thickness somewhat on the anvil with a smooth-faced hammer, taking care to have the edges of equal thickness, and preserving the even surface of the plate as much as possible, constantly annealing so as to avoid brittleness. Having been reduced one fourth of its original substance by forging, it may be taken to the flatting mills and rolled out till it is thin enough for ordinary plate work.

Flatting.—The best form of flatting mill is that shown in Fig. 38. During the process of flatting frequent reference must be made to the gauge (Fig. 39) to see that the plate is of

FIG. 39.

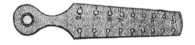

equal thickness all round, the screws holding the two rollers together being regulated accordingly.

Throughout the time of flatting, after every five or six turns through the mill, the plate must be annealed by heating to a dull red colour, as previously mentioned. If a small piece only, this may be done with a blowpipe, but if large it can be more perfectly accomplished with the furnace or forge. For the furnace it must, according to the description in use, be protected from the liability of " sweating," that is, the thin edges and surface becoming partially melted.

Briefly, then, the best results are obtained by compact and careful forging, frequent annealing, and a very gradual and accurate adjustment of the screws of the mill, whereby the rollers are slowly, and at both ends, more nearly approximated, till the plate is finished.

Avoid, especially, straining both gold and mill by jerking and violent rotation of the rollers.

A small quantity of metal may be melted on a block of charcoal and then run into a space formed by another block attached, and having a rim of flattened iron wire interposed, so that

FIG. 40.

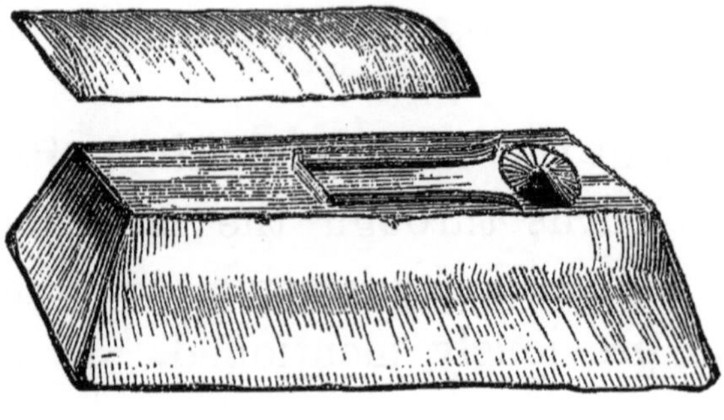

a miniature ingot mould is formed. The charcoal blocks may be embedded in plaster to prevent the hands being liable to injury from the breakage of the charcoal. This plan will be easily understood from the accompanying woodcut (Fig. 40).

The two pieces of charcoal must be tied together with binding wire before melting either with the gas, spirit-lamp, or blow-pipe, is begun.

Making wire requires the gold to be left a good thickness according to the size you require your wire. Then cut off strips with the shears, (Fig. 41), so that they may be square when so

FIG. 41.

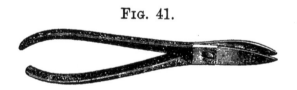

cut off; these must be annealed, then their edges forged with hammer and anvil to take off the sharp borders, and thus reduce the rod to something like a round surface, the metal being constantly annealed throughout; a drawplate, shown in Fig. 42, must be fixed in a strong standard vice and the wire drawn through one hole after another with strong " wire pullers " till it is of the size required for use; it must be constantly annealed and then cooled by passing through a piece of wax; this assists its passage through the holes in the plate. For large

FIG. 42.

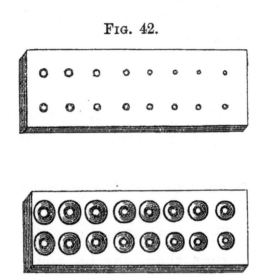

quantities of wire a draw bench is used, by which means a greater amount of force can be applied, but with a small quantity, a little care and steady pulling with the arms will produce very satisfactory results.

Spiral springs.—No one in the present day would think of making their own spiral springs, as they may be obtained of a much better character than home-made ones, at all the depôts, and beyond this a large number of practitioners have dispensed altogether with their application to sets of teeth.

As the appearance of a spring would indicate,

the wire is drawn down thin and then being held firmly at one end the other is attached to a mandrel and gradually spun up till the spiral spring is produced. An instrument in use by dentists some years back, (when they made their own springs,) is shown in Fig. 43, copied from 'Robinson on the Teeth.'

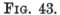

FIG. 43.

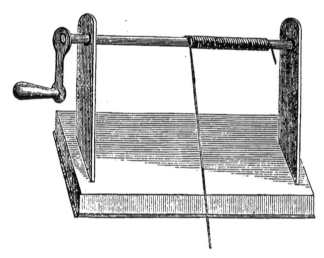

Silver (Ag.). — Equivalent 108; specific gravity from 10·43° to 10·53°; fusing point 107·3°.

Properties.—Exceedingly ductile and malleable, surpassing gold in tenacity, but inferior in this respect to platinum.

Soluble in nitric and sulphuric acids.

Alloys.—Silver is scarcely ever used in the workroom in the pure state on account of its softness ; alloyed with platinum it may be used for wire for certain purposes, but should not be employed as a base for artificial teeth, from the rapidity with which it is acted upon by sulphuretted hydrogen. Silver combines with platinum in varying proportions to form a metal known as Dental alloy ; this is very tough and of a grayish colour. With copper an alloy is formed similar to that of our silver coinage, possessing much greater hardness than pure silver, while it retains its purity of colour. A good proportion is—silver nine parts, copper one part; this is the composition of the silver coinage of the United States, and wears very well. This alloy of silver and copper, however, is of but small interest to the dentist, the more important alloy being with platinum, and this latter having only a very limited application.

Platinum (Pt.).—Equivalent 98·56° ; specific gravity 21·5° ; fusing point, blue heat.

Properties.—In colour it is grayish white, resembling polished steel ; it is harder than silver and has a greater density than any other metal at present known. It can only be melted by the oxy-hydrogen blowpipe and electricity ; no amount of forge or furnace heat will act upon it so that it can be run into an ingot. This metal is exceedingly ductile and malleable when properly tempered and annealed. None of the simple acids have any effect upon it; nitro-muriatic acid, however, dissolves it.

Alloys.—With gold it forms a straw-coloured alloy varying in depth of colour with the quantity of gold used, increasing both the hardness and elasticity of the gold if the latter be in excess; hence the use of platinum in gold intended for spring wire, clasps, &c.

Platinum is best used in the pure state—if at all—for plates for artificial teeth, as it then keeps a good colour and retains its polish very well. Pure gold must be used as a solder if the platinum be pure.

SECTION VI

MAKING GOLD PLATES FOR PARTIAL AND FULL DENTURES

THE models having been prepared in accordance with the directions already given, a pattern must be cut out in thin sheet lead, so that on being applied to the model it perfectly covers every part that is to be fitted with a plate; this being removed, is flattened out carefully and placed upon a sheet of gold of the requisite thickness, and the outline traced with a sharp-pointed instrument or pencil. The size of the plate will vary according to the position of the tooth or teeth to be replaced, and according as to whether it is to be retained by clasps or bands around the other teeth or by suction. I shall first treat of cases held in the mouth by clasps and bands. If there is an opening between the bicuspid and molar on either side, the plate should be carried back so that a support may be fitted around the latter, taking

it for granted that an artificial tooth is required
at the anterior part of the mouth. For such
an arrangement the plate may be made of the
form shown in Fig. 44, or if the covering of

FIG. 44.

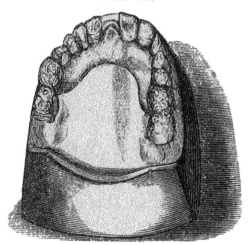

the palate produces discomfort it may be
narrowed in front and a bridge of metal carried
across from molar to molar, as shown in Fig.
45 ; this leaves all that part of the mouth
quite clear against which the tongue principally
presses in speech and deglutition. It is very
important in single tooth cases, especially, that
they should fit with great firmness and depend
for their support upon bands attached to very
sound teeth. If from any cause bands cannot
be adjusted to the first molars, the second
bicuspids may be used, but in some patients'

Fig. 45.

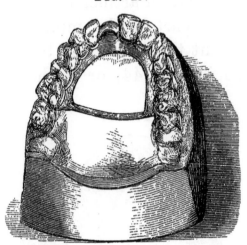

mouths there is a liability of the clasp showing
when the teeth are displayed, as in laughter.

These remarks as to the clasps apply to all
cases where any of the eight anterior teeth are
required.   The plan suggested of cutting out
the central portion of the plate, thus leaving
the palate exposed, may also be adopted for
these cases.

The plate having been cut out according to
pattern by means of the shears and nippers
shown in Figs. 46 and 47 and the situation of
the clasps decided on, the next step is "striking
up ;" this is accomplished by placing the plate
between the die and counter die and giving it
one or two steady blows with a flat-faced
hammer weighing about six or seven pounds,
the weight of the hammer varying according to

the strength of the workman. The gold must have been struck and bent somewhat into shape,

FIG. 46.

FIG. 47.

FIG. 48.

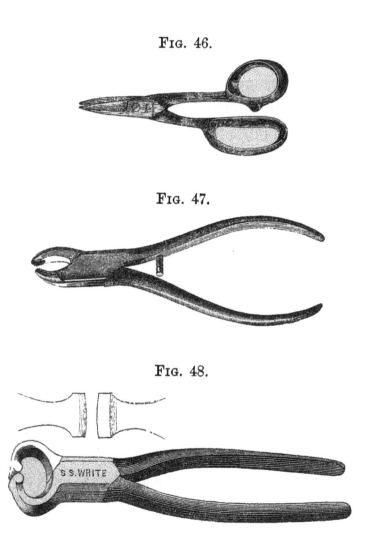

first, on the zinc model with the aid of a mallet of wood or horn and the pliers for this purpose (Fig. 48). If the teeth in the mouth are very long they may be cut down (after the model is dipped in lead) to within one eighth of an inch from the gum; this will facilitate the process of striking up, and the teeth having been cut down after the counter die is taken admits of more pressure being brought directly upon the plate instead of upon the crown of the teeth. During the process of fitting the plate it will become necessary to frequently anneal it, in order that it may not become cracked and brittle from the hardening; previously to annealing it is very important to bear in mind that it should always be placed for five or ten minutes in dilute hydrochloric acid or boiled in dilute acid, and afterwards well brushed with pumice powder and water, so as to remove all particles of lead or zinc that may have adhered to the surface; these, if not removed before annealing, injure the quality of the plate.

By the aid of the blowpipe or furnace it should then be brought to a dull red heat.

One model and counter die will scarcely suffice to make a plate fit the plaster model and mouth perfectly, there should always be a second set ready for use; and in the event of the markings on the palate being very prominent, or the plate having to fit over stumps, it is even well

to use a third zinc model and lead. The fit of
the plate round the necks of the remaining teeth
should be very accurate, to attain this end
many use chasing punches of the form shown
in Fig. 49. Others again prefer only to trust

FIG. 49.

to the fit obtained by the striking up. Before
the final swaging the plate must be reduced to
the size it is to assume in the finished state.
This can be done with the file, the palatine
border of the plate being finished off with a
bevelled or scissor edge, and the other portions
so as to present no rough edges to the tongue.
If teeth are to be mounted on the gum, then the
plate must be cut away in a scalloped form,
corresponding with the outlines of the face of
the teeth, the teeth must, however, slightly
overlap the border so that none of the plate

may be seen when in the mouth.   It is scarcely necessary to point out that during the process of making the plate any fractures that may have taken place in it must be repaired with solder, and, if necessary, a small strip of gold put across the breakage to act as a brace; any parts, also, that from their position will be subjected in the mouth to great strain, must be strengthened either by doubling the plate at this point, or by soldering on a strip of half round wire, striking it up with the plate before fixing, so as to obtain perfect apposition of the two.   When the narrow strip of plate is carried across the arch of the palate, it should be increased in substance carefully, so as to withstand the pressure that may be applied in putting it into and removing it from the mouth. When *in situ* there is but slight strain upon it, resting as it does between two fixed points on a solid base.   It is particularly important to well sustain those parts of the plate that run forward to carry only a single tooth, as these are peculiarly liable to breakage, and have to resist great force when the teeth are closed in the natural bite during mastication.

Bands and clasps.—The plate completed, is ready for trying in the mouth; any alterations that are necessary must now be made before fitting the bands. If its adaptation to the mouth is perfect we may at once proceed to make the clasps. Here we enter upon a much debated topic, for there are many very diverse opinions as to the proper way of making and arranging them. The plan most generally adopted is to take a strip of gold (alloyed with platinum is best), of a suitable width, and with the hand pliers (Fig. 50) adjust it to the tooth, so that the surfaces of the two are in perfect apposition; the band is then fitted carefully to the plate, and united as I shall presently describe.

FIG. 50.

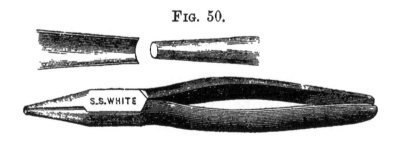

Dr Spalding, of the United States, has invented a form of band called the " Standard " clasp, that allows the neck of the tooth to be exposed, thus enabling the tongue and saliva to clear away any particles of food that might accumulate. The band is fitted as just described, but it is not allowed to rest upon the gum, it is supported midway between the neck

of the tooth and the grinding surface by means
of standards, which, running up from the plate
(itself cut clear of the tooth), supports the band.
This plan will be more readily understood by
reference to the accompanying sketch (Fig. 51).

FIG. 51.

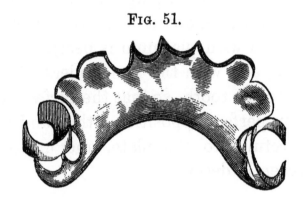

The standards and bands should both be of the
same width, and made of platinized gold.   This
plan is, however, open to the objection that the
gum will very probably become hypertrophied,
and grow through the spaces left in the plate,
and thus produce a more mischievous condition
than if ordinary clasps had been used.

Still a third, and in my own opinion in many
respects the best way of applying bands to
molar teeth, is to take a strip of platinum very
thin and soft, and applying this to the tooth,
press it carefully with a burnishing instrument
into all the inequalities, so that it perfectly embraces the tooth from the neck to the crown;

remove this very carefully, and place in the open centre of it a mixture of plaster and sand or plaster and asbestos (2 parts plaster, 1 part sand or asbestos). As soon as it is thoroughly dry, brush over the exposed surface with borax and water, and put on some small pieces of plate gold, and then applying a good solid flame with the blowpipe, fuse the gold evenly over the surface of the platina, repeat this till you have the substance of the band rather thicker than an ordinary clasp; it may, after this, be filed down to a suitable form like a common band, we thus get the most perfect adaptation, with great strength and elasticity.

It is generally a matter of difficulty to retain the clasps in their right position when removing them from the model or mouth after they have been fitted to each other. If the plate and bands attached can be removed easily on account of the sides of the teeth being perpendicular, then it is only necessary to see that you have the clasps attached to the plate securely before attempting removal; this may be done in several ways: first, and most commonly, by means of resin and wax applied round the neck of the band where it joins the plate; secondly, by using sealing wax instead of the former substance, which possesses the advantage of greater hardness, and breaks with a clean fracture instead of bending like resin and wax ; thirdly, by coating over with a solution of soap the surface of the model near the plate, and then pouring on plaster and sand, and when it is set hard removing, if possible, with the plate and bands attached ; if not, adjusting them to it afterwards and then resting the under surface of the plate and the clasps in a mass of the plaster compound, and when hardened removing the upper and first cast that was made to give their relative positions ; this is a little trouble-some, but a very certain mode of procedure. The same may be done in the mouth ; fit them into their places and then take an impression extending well beyond the plate, in either wax or plaster of Paris. . They will be tolerably certain to come away with the tray ; if they do not they can easily be removed and put into their proper place in the cast. The impression can now be cast, not, however, with plaster only, but with a mixture of plaster and asbestos; we then obtain a model with the plate and clasps in position, so that we may warm up in the oven and proceed to solder at once with the most perfect assurance that they cannot have shifted.

When by one or other of the preceding

methods the bands and plates are safely imbedded ready for soldering, the surface must be
carefully cleaned of wax if it has been used or
any particles of plaster ; the joints coated with
borax and water, and small pieces of solder put
on. As soon as the furnace has brought the
case up to a good red heat it may be soldered
by the blowpipe. After cooling down (not too
rapidly) and "pickling," trim up with a file and
scorper, and the plate is ready for mounting
the teeth on. It is, however, a wise precaution
to again try it in the mouth to see that the
bands are correct.

For lower plates the proceeding is nearly the
same as for the upper, with the obvious difference that they do not require support to be
given them, but steadiness ; this may be done
by a couple of clasps round the bicuspids whenever it is possible, or clips passing between
them. These teeth being the most favorable
for applying bands, this rule applies with
equal force whether the teeth have to be replaced at either the anterior or posterior part
of the mouth.

The piece must always be strengthened with
a double thickness of gold at the most central
part, as from the formation of the lower jaw
there is no mechanical advantage to be gained,

such as we have in the flat palate of the upper maxilla, where a comparatively thin plate will suffice.   Three different forms of lower plates are shown in Figs. 52, 53, and 54.

For lower cases, where there is much loose mucous membrane, it is well to build up the model a little, so that the edge of the plate may present a rounded border ; this is done by adding some thin plaster or resin and wax to the model before casting in metal.

Instead of this plan being adopted, thin wire may be soldered on the upper edge of the plate, and the lower edge filed up to it so as to give the same result.

Suction plates.—A plan that is frequently adopted for retaining upper dentures in their place is that of atmospheric pressure or suction ; by this method all fastenings to the natural teeth are avoided ; the plate is extended over a considerable surface of the hard palate, and the pressure of the air against its lower surface is sufficient if it be accurately fitted to retain the plate firmly in its proper position ; for this mode of attachment the impression should always be taken in plaster of Paris, and great care be taken to obtain a perfect adaptation of the plate to the mouth.

Air chambers are formed occasionally in

FIG. 52.

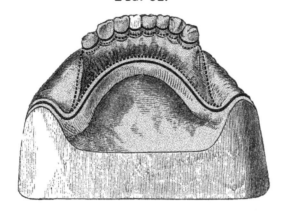

FIG. 53.

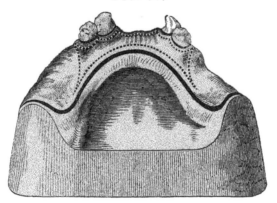

FIG. 54.

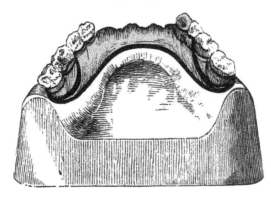

the plates for the purpose of increasing the suction, but from my own experience pieces as a rule hold up quite as well if not better without them.

To make a suction chamber, either cut out a depression, oval or shield-shaped, in the plaster impression before casting the model, or form with plaster or wax an elevation of the required form on the palatine surface of the plaster model before making a metal cast ; the plate is struck up to this, and the sharp angles obtained by chasing round with a suitably shaped punch. In the preceding cuts are shown air chambers of the various forms in most common use, Figs. 55, 56, and 57. They admit, of course, of great variety in form, according to the nature of the case under treatment.

FIG. 55.

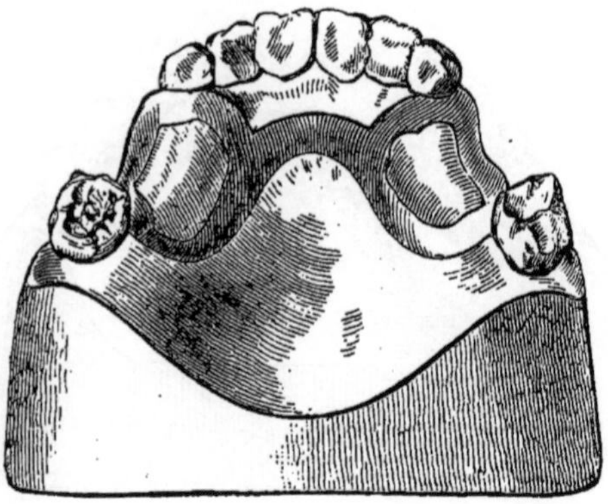

FIG. 56.

FIG 57.

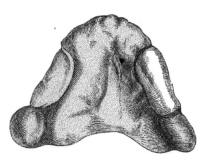
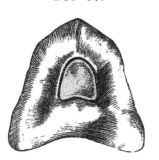

Making plates for complete upper dentures.— Cut out the pattern in thin sheet lead as for a partial plate; if it is to be retained in the mouth by suction, let it not only invest entirely the alveolar ridge, but also cover completely the hard palate; if, on the other hand, it is to be supported by spiral springs, the plate need not extend so far over the palate, but may assume the form of a horseshoe for its palatine outline. Having been well annealed, it may be bent with the pliers and beaten into shape with the mallet till it will rest upon the model with something approaching the finished form. Though this part of the process takes but few words to describe, it requires some time and skill to accomplish, the principal difficulty arising from the "buckling" of the plate bending it over upon itself in the most awkward places, and tending to a displacement from the position you desire it to occupy. It is especially apt to slip backwards or forwards on the zinc model. A very useful and simple contrivance to avoid this has been devised by Dr Kurras, of New York. The form is shown in Fig. 58. The

FIG. 58.

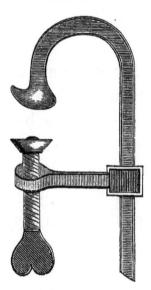

metal die with the plate on it is placed near the edge of the work board; the clamp is applied to the central portion of the palate (protecting the plate by some linen, or two or three folds of brown packing paper) and the screw being tightened underneath the bench, the plate is held firmly in position, while with the mallet the overlaps are brought into contact with the alveolar ridge. If this descends perpendicularly, or is undercut at all, the plate will double upon itself. V-shaped portions must be cut out, allowing only sufficient for the one cut edge to overlap the other; they may afterwards be bevelled off on the reverse sides of the edges, so as to leave a smoother surface when they are soldered up. The plate being now roughly bent into shape, is ready for striking up; this is done as with partial cases by placing it between the die and counter die, and giving it a succession of steady blows with a heavy hammer.

Another plan is to apply the blow by an arrangement somewhat like a guillotine, in which a heavy weight retained between two upright bars is allowed to fall directly upon the die; and ensure an evenly distributed blow; it is open to the objection, however, of not being so easily regulated as when a hammer is used with the hand.

If an air chamber is introduced into the plate it may be made in the same way as for a partial denture; there is, however, another variety of chamber that is only well suited to complete dentures; this is known as Cleveland's, and its construction is thus described by Dr Richardson; an ordinary plate with chamber struck up, is first made, and the chamber cut out.

A thin sheet of wax, or a layer of plaster, is then placed upon the lingual side of the plate, extending from two to three or four lines from the edges of the orifice in the main edge; a thin, retreating edge is given to the wax or plaster at the outer borders, making it continuous with the surface of the plate. The plate with the wax attached may now either be tacked to the model with softened wax along its outer borders, and shaped in such a way as to permit the model and plate to be withdrawn from the sand, and a mould of the parts taken in the ordinary way, and from this a die and counter; or an impression in wax or plaster may be taken of the lingual face of the plate and wax, and afterwards a model, die, and counter. With the latter, a second plate, covering nearly or quite all of the palatal concavity is swaged, and when this is applied to the main plate over the cut chamber, and united by soldering, a space, equal to the thickness of the wax, or plaster placed on the primary plate, will be found to exist between the two lamina. Fig. 59 exhibits a transverse section of the two plates, disclosing the space between them, and also the opening through the gum plate into the cavity. Before soldering on the duplicate plate, a half-round wire should be soldered around the opening in the palatal plate on its lingual side, to protect the soft tissues of the mouth from injury when drawn in as the air is exhausted from the chamber; or, what is preferable, this form of cavity may be converted, practically, into what is known as "Gilbert's chamber" (which is the central swaged chamber before described), by filling in the space between the two plates with some impervious substance, as Hill's filling, or an amalgam of gold, the excess of mercury being driven off by

FIG. 59.

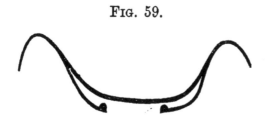

heat. In the construction of continuous gum work, the interspace may be filled in with gum body. The advantages of these double plates are, a greatly increased strength imparted to the base, a diminished liability of warping in the process of soldering, a smoother surface presented to the tongue, and a more decidedly angular form of the chamber.

It is occasionally useful to solder a thin wire on the palatal surface of the plate following the inner border of the alveolar ridge, and crossing the palate about one eighth of an inch from the free border of the plate. A plate prepared in this way will generally have remarkably good suction, and hold up very firmly, and as the wire ridge makes for itself a depression in the soft tissues of the hard palate, the amount of lateral movement (of which most plates are capable) will be very much reduced.

It is desirable occasionally to solder a rim of wire or plate round the alveolar border of a full upper denture to present a rounded surface in the mouth, and thus avoid cutting into the mucous membrane; this is done by bending the wire or strip of plate to the proper form and then fixing with binding wire to hold it in position while soldering.

Making a plate for complete lower denture. —This process is for the most part the same as for an upper plate.

It is very necessary, however, that the metal should be thicker and more elastic; it must also be strengthened by a rim of plate covering the alveolar ridge, and thin wire should be soldered all round if possible, but in any case on its lingual border. Some prefer using a thin plate first and then adding a second thick layer of metal to its external surface, thus avoiding the use of the wire border and producing a very strong serviceable base for the denture.

Whether the wire and strengthener together or separately are used, the piece must be well swaged afterwards to counteract the warping that generally takes place from the contraction during soldering. One other plan yet remains to be mentioned, that is, to use a single thick plate and turn up the edges and fill in the depression with good solder, and thus obtain a rounded border. The wire I consider, however, the best mode to adopt. The general form of plate for a full lower denture is shown in Fig. 60.

FIG. 60.

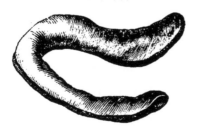

Obtaining the bite for a partial denture.— This may be done in three different ways. The first plan is to have a model of both the upper and lower jaws.

When the plate is made cover those spaces that are to be filled up with artificial teeth, with strips of tough wax (one formula recommended consists of two ounces of gum mastic to a pound of wax, and one ounce of Spanish whiting; this has to be melted, and the other ingredients added in a fine state of division).

The wax is made to adhere firmly by slightly warming the plate over the spirit lamp. As soon as the wax is trimmed up neatly it may be placed in the mouth and the patient directed to close the jaws in the usual way. Great care must be taken to see that this is done; as a rule patients will shut the jaws in any possible manner rather than that which is normal; it is therefore wise to repeat the process several times to see that each " bite " corresponds. If the rim of wax has been left full above the level of the surrounding teeth in the model, we shall find when the plate is removed from the mouth that the points of antagonism are accurately marked on the wax. Being replaced on the model, the opposing jaw in the plaster cast can be adjusted to the impression of the natural teeth in the wax, and held in this relation, a permanent articulation can be made. The back surfaces of the models must be coated with soap and then mixing some plaster very stiff, place the models in it, the plaster resting on a smooth surface, such as marble or glass, with a sheet of thin paper interposed to prevent adhesion; the result that will be obtained is shown in Fig. 61.

FIG. 61.

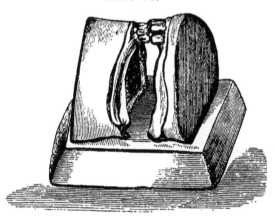

The second form of articulation is known as a hawksbill bite: to obtain this you act in precisely the same way as for the last, only instead of having a model of the opposing jaw, you use the impression left on the wax instead, and by filling in with plaster, obtain a model from it, of those teeth only that come into contact with the artificial denture. The form thus obtained is shown in Fig. 62. Before pouring the plaster over the wax the operator must be careful to fill in the centre of the model with paper, to avoid an excess of plaster here, and at the same time make either crucial grooves or depressions on the back of the

FIG. 62

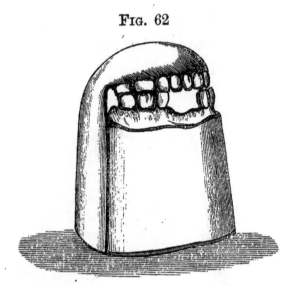

model as an indication for the after-adjustment of the two parts of the bite.

A modification of the last form of bite is made by extending the back of the model thus, Fig. 63 ;

FIG. 63.

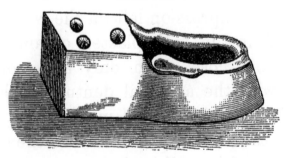

and putting on the wax bite, proceeding as in the last case, only making the upper and posterior surfaces flat, so that the articulated models

will stand either way, as seen in Figs. 64
and 65.

FIG. 64.

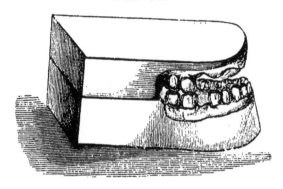

FIG. 65.

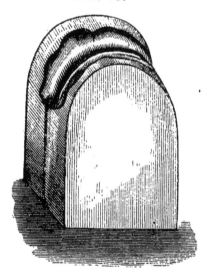

By binding them together with a broad
elastic band, we obtain a very convenient working bite.

If the front teeth of the upper jaw have to be
replaced, then the central and horizontal lines of

the mouth must be obtained when taking the bite. This can easily be done by marking the wax crucially with a sharp instrument, and afterwards marking the models to correspond before displacing the wax.

Obtaining the bite for an entire upper and lower denture.—This is very difficult to do with certainty, unless the patient has an old artificial case by which you may be assisted. It is scarcely possible to get the bite right the first time, so that it is wiser to carefully watch the relative position of the jaws when the patient is not conscious of your observation; then taking a bite as nearly accurate as you can, mount up artificial blocks of wax strengthened with wire and without any teeth attached, and by their use get a more certain closure of the jaws. It is sometimes advisable also to watch for the position of the jaws during the act of swallowing, taking care to divert the attention of the patient at the time. Of two "bites" taken together, but differing in the position of the lower jaw, it will always be safer to choose that in which the inferior maxilla is most retracted, since as the backward movement of the jaw is very limited, you have under these circumstances the least liability to derangement of the normal position of the jaws. It is a very good plan to load the lower in the centre of the wax with strips of lead so that it may not move about in the mouth; this, of course, must not be done with the upper.

Spiral springs may occasionally be used with advantage in taking a "bite," as they keep the upper and lower trial plates in good position, and by offering some slight opposition to the closure of the jaws probably induce a more natural movement of the inferior maxilla than if they were not used.

I believe, from my own experience, it is only possible to get a good bite after you have all the teeth mounted on the plates with cement; you can then fairly judge of the effect produced by any malposition, which you cannot do with a block of wax alone. The depth of the bite should be such that with the mouth in a state of repose, the margins of the lips touch without any muscular action whatever; this, I think, will be found in all normal cases, a sound guide.

The two models may be arranged in either of the forms of bite already described, or they may be fitted up in an adjustable articulator, as shown in Fig. 66.

This articulator is recommended as having all the necessary movements for obtaining a cor-

FIG. 66.

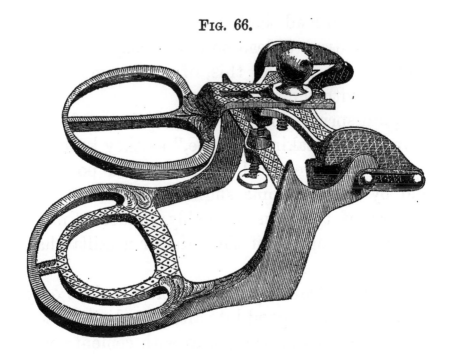

rect articulation of artificial dentures. The
lower plate is moulded from the lower jaw, and
moves on cone-shaped pivots in V-shaped
grooves (without hinges), being retained in
position by elastic-rubber bands or rings. A
backward, forward, and lateral motion is provided for, corresponding with the movements
of the natural jaw, by which the arrangement
of the denture can be practically tested without
disturbing the articulation. The upper plate
has a backward and forward movement of two
inches, and may be retained at any point by
the set screw. The upper plate has a double
bend, so that when reversed from the position

shown in the cut an increase of one inch in
the space is obtained between the plates, allowing for both upper and lower dentures.

Another form, simpler in structure, is shown
in Fig. 67. This is made of brass, having a

FIG. 67.

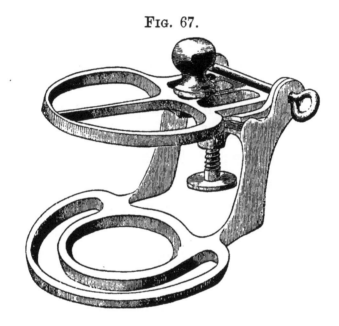

screw and hinge, whereby it can be adjusted
at any desired angle; the top plate can be
thrown right back and the set screw allows
the plate to slide either backwards or forwards.

SECTION VII

ON THE VARIOUS FORMS OF PORCELAIN USED IN MECHANICAL DENTISTRY

SCARCELY any dental surgeon in the present day would think of making his own mineral teeth and blocks; at the same time it is desirable that some account of the process by which they are prepared by our large dental manufacturers should be given; I must, however, warn the reader that it is not to be taken as an accurate description of the actual work carried on by them; as in this country at any rate they guard the secrets of their tooth factories with a most religious jealousy. We know, however, sufficient to form a tolerably clear idea of the methods by which our present make of mineral teeth are prepared. We shall speak first of single teeth; then of sectional blocks with mineral gum attached; and, lastly, as an associate process, of continuous gum work.

Composition.—Some makers' teeth are of the same composition throughout; others, however, have a less dense but stronger material for the body of the tooth, and a transparent but somewhat brittle preparation as an enamel or outer covering.

The materials used are kaolin (white clay), silex, and felspar; none of these minerals are fusible at a low temperature, nor, when fused, are they acted upon by acids, hence their extreme utility for artificial teeth. The various colours and shades are imparted by means of metallic oxides in a fine state of division, of which I shall presently give an account.

The materials having been prepared very carefully so as to reduce them to a complete powder, are weighed off in their relative proportions and then made into a paste by the addition of distilled or rain water. Brass or copper moulds are used for forming the teeth in, consisting of two portions, one in which is the impress of the tooth and the other which represents the back of the tooth, and is pierced with two fine holes, opposite each impression through which the platina pins are passed. The paste for the body is pressed into these moulds, and the pins put in through the openings on the upper plate. A few taps of the hammer will dislodge them from the mould when dry, and they are then taken out and placed on a fire-clay slide and heated to a bright red; as soon as they are sufficiently cool they are trimmed up carefully and all roughness or inequality removed, and placed again on the slide with the face upwards (the pins resting in a grove and the slide being sprinkled with silex).

The enamel is now very carefully and evenly applied with a brush, the various tints being arranged on the face of the tooth in accordance with the result desired. They are again dried and then introduced into the furnace.

The great perfection to which this branch of manufacture has attained during the last few years is very surprising, but it can be easily understood when we consider the enormous sale that has been created with the supply, and the very potent stimulus that has thus been given to enterprise, and invention, so as to produce the most perfect results.

It is owing to the numberless inventions and varieties of procedure, in connexion with this department, that such jealousy is induced on the part of the makers in guarding the secrets of their laboratories.

American authors publish a large number of recipes for the enamel and body of teeth, but whether they are identical with those in use by

American tooth-makers we have no means of ascertaining ; from the fact, however, that many American dental surgeons prepare their own sectional blocks, they are sufficient for our present purpose.

According to Harris, a good compound for single teeth consists in the following :

Body.

Spar	. . . .	10 oz.
Silex	. . . .	1 „
Kaolin .	. . .	2 dwts.
Titanium	. . .	1 „

Enamel.

Spar	. . . .	1 oz.
Silex	. . . .	3 grs.
Flint glass	. . .	2 „
Titanium	. . .	1 „
Platina sponge	. .	3 „

These will produce ordinary tints for the teeth ; they are, however, capable of infinite variety by the use of one or other of the following metals or metallic oxides, alone or in combination, as the case may require.

*Metals and their oxides.**	*Colours produced.*
Gold in a state of minute division	. Rose red.
Oxide of gold	. Bright rose red.
Platina sponge and filings . .	. Grayish blue.

* Richardson's ' Mechanical Dentistry.'

Metals and their oxides.					*Colours produced.*
Oxide of titanium	.	.	.	.	Bright yellow.
Purple of cassius	.	.	.	.	Rose purple.
Oxide of uranium	.	.	.	.	Greenish yellow.
Oxide of manganese	.	.	.	.	Purple.
Oxide of cobalt	.	.	.	.	Bright blue.
Oxide of silver	.	.	.	.	Lemon yellow.
Oxide of zinc	.	.	.	.	Lemon yellow.

Sectional blocks are made by striking up a gold plate first with a rim round the alveolar ridge, then modelling up with the body, of which the various compounds are given further on. Being set up in solid blocks they are allowed to dry and then trimmed up and carved with a steel instrument or penknife into the shape the teeth are to assume, great care being taken to avoid crumbling when in this dry state ; the platina pins are then introduced, the blocks being placed on the furnace slides resting on their lower border so as only to let the part that fits the plate come into contact with the pulverized silex with which the slide is covered. These blocks are made usually in three sections, if for an entire denture; one for the four incisors and canines, and two for the bicuspids and molars, consisting of two bicuspids and two molars to each section.

Composition for body of block teeth.

1. Delaware spar   .   .   .   . 12 oz.
   Silex   .   .   .   .   . 2 oz. 8 dwts.
   Kaolin .   .   .   .   . 7½ dwts.
   Titanium   .   .   .   . 18 to 36 grs.

2. Delaware spar   .   .   .   . 16 oz.
   Silex   .   .   .   .   . 3½ ,,
   Kaolin .   .   .   .   . ½ ,,
   Titanium   .   .   .   . 20 to 60 grs.

3. Delaware spar   .   .   .   . 12 oz.
   Silex   .   .   .   .   . 2 oz. 8 dwts.
   Kaolin .   .   .   .   . 12 dwts.
   Titanium   .   .   .   . 24 grs.

4. Delaware spar   .   .   .   . 8 oz.
   Silex   .   .   .   .   . 1½ ,,
   Kaolin .   .   .   .   . 4 dwts.
   Titanium   .   .   .   . 22 grs.

5. Delaware spar   .   .   .   . 2 oz.
   Silex   .   .   .   .   . 8 dwts.
   Kaolin .   .   .   .   . 2 ,,
   Titanium   .   .   .   . 4 grs.

Grayish-blue enamel for porcelain block teeth.

1. Spar   .   .   .   .   .   . 2 oz.
   Platina sponge   .   .   . ¼ gr.
   Oxide of gold   .   .   . ½ ,,

2. Spar   .   .   .   .   .   . 2 oz.
   Platina sponge   .   .   . ¼ gr.
   Oxide of gold   .   .   . ½ ,,

3. Spar   .   .   .   .   .   . 2 oz.
   Platina sponge   .   .   . ¾ gr.
   Oxide of gold   .   .   . ½ ,,

4. Spar . . . . . . 2 oz.
   Flux . . . . . . 24 grs.
   Platina sponge . . . . ½ gr.

Yellow enamel for porcelain block teeth.

1. Spar . . . . . . 2 oz.
   Titanium . . . . . 10 grs.
   Platina sponge . . . . ½ gr.
   Oxide of gold . . . . ½ „

2. Spar . . . . . . 2 oz.
   Titanium . . . . . 14 grs.
   Platina sponge . . . . ½ gr.
   Oxide of gold . . . . ½ „

3. Spar . . . . . . 2 oz.
   Titanium . . . . . 16 grs.
   Platina sponge . . . . ½ gr.
   Oxide of gold . . . . ½ „

4. Spar . . . . . . 2 oz.
   Flux . . . . . . 20 grs.
   Titanium . . . . . 10 „

Grayish-blue enamel for porcelain block teeth.

1. Spar . . . . . . 1 oz.
   Blue frit . . . . . 5 grs.

2. Spar . . . . . . 1 oz.
   Yellow frit . . . . 4 grs.
   Gold mixture . . . . 10 „

Composition and preparation of gum enamels.

1. Gum frit, No. 1 . . . . 3 dwts.
   Spar . . . . . . 9 to 12 dwts.

2 Gum frit, No. 2 . . . . 3 dwts.
   Spar . . . . . . 3 to 18 dwts.

Boston spar is preferred on account of its greater fusibility. Flux is composed of—

Silex	4 oz.
Borax	1 „
Sal tartar . . .	1 „

These are ground to an impalpable powder and packed in the bottom of a clean, light-coloured crucible. A piece of fire-clay slab is then fitted into the top of the crucible and luted with kaolin clay.

It is then exposed to the heat of a furnace until completely fused, when it is removed, and as soon as it is cold the crucible is broken, all foreign particles or discoloured portions thoroughly removed, and the remainder well pulverized. Blue frit is composed of—

Spar	$\frac{1}{2}$ oz.
Platina sponge . .	4 dwts.

Powder very finely, make up into a ball with water, and fuse very slightly upon a slide in a furnace. It must then be plunged into water while hot, and when dry, finely pulverized.

Yellow frit is made by mixing intimately $\frac{1}{2}$ oz. of spar with two dwts. of titanium and heating as above.

Gold mixture is made by dissolving 8 grains of pure gold in aqua regia, then stirring in $12\frac{1}{2}$ dwts. of very finely pulverized spar. When nearly dry it is formed into a ball, and fused upon a slide, and then coarsely pulverized.

Continuous gum work, though very useful and beautiful, requires great care, special conveniences, and considerable experience to produce in a satisfactory state, and when finished to the delight of the dental surgeon, is not appreciated by the patient for whom it has been prepared, chiefly on account of its extreme weight.   These remarks apply especially to this country, where the knowledge of the patient is far behind the resources and capabilities of the dental practitioner ; hence dentures of continuous gum work are comparatively rarely made here.   In the United States, however, it is much more in fashion, in part owing, probably, to its having been invented there, partly, also, from the greater willingness of American patients to put up with personal inconvenience, and even discomfort for a time, in order to obtain a perfect result.

To Dr Allen is given the credit of this invention.   I shall, therefore, give a description of the process in the Doctor's own words as it appears in Dr Richardson's work.

Dr Allen's Modes of Practice.—The following descriptions, contributed by Dr Allen, embrace a clear and concise account of the manipulations at present practised by him in the construction of artificial dentures, with continuous gums.

" The plate or base is formed of platinum, or platinum and iridium. The plate being properly fitted to the mouth, and wax placed upon it for the bite, as in ordinary plate work, the teeth are arranged thereon, with special reference to the requirements of the case. They are then covered with a thin coating of plaster mixed with water to the consistence of cream. After this has become firmly set, another mixture of plaster and asbestos with water, somewhat thicker or more plastic than the first, is placed round on the outside of the previous covering and the plate. A convenient way of applying the second covering is to turn the mixture out of the vessel upon a piece of tin, say four or five inches square, thus forming a cone upon which the plate with the teeth upward, is pressed gently down until within an inch or less from the tin. Then with a spatula the mixture is brought up over the teeth, forming an investient that will not crack in the process of soldering. Sand may be used with the plaster for this purpose, but I think asbestos preferable.

" When the covering has become sufficiently

hard the wax is removed, and a rim of platinum
is then fitted to the lingual side of the teeth,
below the pins, and to the base plate. The
pins in the teeth are then bent down upon the
rim, and soldered with pure gold, or a mixture
of gold and platinum, at the same time the rim
is soldered to the plate. This rim, which forms
the lining for the teeth, is usually about the
thickness of the plate upon which they are set,
say 28 to 30;* but should the case require
more than ordinary strength, a double or triple
thickness of rim should be used. This may
become necessary in cases where the natural
molar teeth are standing firmly in the opposite
jaw, and antagonise with the artificial piece, or
where from any cause, an undue strain is brought
to bear upon the artificial teeth. To attain successful results, the dentist must take into consideration all the circumstances or conditions
of each particular case, and then exercise his
best judgment in executing the work.

"In soldering platinum with pure gold, flat
surfaces of this metal should be brought in
positive contact, in order to become firmly
united. Therefore, in mounting teeth upon
a plate of this kind, the backing or inside
rim should be a little wider than the distance

* American gauge.

between the pins in the teeth and the plate, say from an eighth to a fourth of an inch. This extra width of rim should be bent at right angles along the base of the teeth so as to admit of being pressed down upon the plate after the rim is adjusted to the teeth, and the pins bent down firmly upon it. In this way flat surfaces of the rim and plate are brought together and soldered. The pins in the teeth are also soldered to the rim at the same time. When the parts are thus united, they will remain so during the subsequent bakings; but if the edge of the rim only is fitted to the plate and soldered like gold or silver work, the subsequent heatings for baking the body and gum will cause the gold to become absorbed in the platinum, and leave the joints not united. It may be asked why not use common gold solder for this style of work? Answer, because the alloy in the solder will greatly injure the colour of the gum enamel in baking. Copper alloy will turn it to a greenish shade, and silver will give it a yellow tinge. Although pure gold requires more intense heat to melt it (being about two thousand degrees), than ordinary gold solder, yet when melted it flows much more freely than the latter. The best way to solder the teeth upon platinum plate is, to place small pieces of gold upon the

joints or parts to be soldered, with wet ground
borax, and then slowly introduce the piece with
the investient into a heated muffle, and bring the
whole mass up to a red heat ; then withdraw it
from the furnace, and bring it quickly under
the blow-pipe to flow the gold.   In this way
the teeth do not become etched, as they are
liable to be if the soldering is done in the
furnace.

" The piece being soldered and cooled, the
covering is removed from the teeth, taking care
to preserve the base unbroken for the plate to
sit upon during the subsequent bakings of the
body and gum enamel.

" All particles of plaster or other foreign
matter should be removed from the teeth and
plate by thoroughly washing and brushing them.
It is well to immerse the piece for a short time
in sulphuric acid, after which rinse and brush it
well with water.   This done, a colourless
mineral compound, called the body, is applied
in a plastic state (with spatulas or small in-
instruments for the purpose) to the teeth and
plate.   It is then carved to represent the gum,
roof and ruga of the mouth, taking care to keep
the crowns of the teeth well defined.   The
piece is then placed on the base upon which it
was soldered and set upon a slide on the apron

in front of one of the upper muffles of the
heated furnace,—and every eight or ten minutes
it should be moved forward into the muffle, say
two or four inches each time, until the piece
shall have passed the centre of the same, which
should be at a red heat.   It is then withdrawn
and passed into a lower muffle where the heat
is greater, in which the body soon becomes
semi-vitrified, which is sufficient for the first
bake.   It is then taken out and (together with
the slide on which it was baked) placed in a
cooling muffle, the mouth of which should be
closed to prevent the change of temperature
from being too rapid, and causing the teeth to
become brittle.   When the piece is sufficiently
cool to handle, a second application of body is
made for the purpose of repairing any defects
that may have occurred in the baking; this
done, the piece is again introduced as before
into the upper muffle, then in the lower,
allowing the second bake to become a little
harder than the first, but not so much as to
appear glossy.   It is then withdrawn, and
cooled as described above.

" A flesh-coloured compound is then applied,
which is called the gum enamel.   This is also
made plastic with water, and a thin coating is
put over the body, and closely packed and

carved around the teeth with small instruments made for the purpose,—still taking care to keep the crowns of the teeth clean and well defined. Small camel's-hair brushes are used wet with water, to cause the gum enamel and also the body to settle more closely around the necks of the teeth; other brushes are also used dry to remove all particles of body, gum, or other substances from the crowns of the teeth.

"After the application of the gum enamel the piece is again subjected to the heat of the furnace as described for baking the body, with this difference:—the heat should be a little greater than for either of the preceding bakes. It should be a strong, sharp heat, in order to produce a smooth glossy appearance which is required for the enamel. These different degrees of heat for the first, second and third bakings should be carefully observed for the purpose of getting an even temper in the piece, and thereby preventing it from crazing or cracking in cooling.

"The enamel being thoroughly fused, the piece is withdrawn from the heated muffle, and passed into another, outside of the furnace. This muffle should be made quite hot before the denture is placed in it, in order to prolong the cooling process; for if the piece is cooled too rapidly, it is rendered more fragile. It is well to let the case remain in the cooling muffle, with the mouth of it closed, several hours before exposing it to the air. By baking just at night, the piece will be in proper condition to finish up the next morning.

"The finishing process consists simply in smoothing and polishing the plate, and burnishing the rim. It is then ready to be adjusted to the mouth. In baking, great care is necessary to prevent the piece from becoming gassed. This can be avoided by allowing the gas to escape entirely from the burning coal or coke in the furnace before the piece is introduced into the muffle. The presence of gas is indicated by the blue flame escaping from the coal. When the fire becomes clear, it is then safe to introduce the case to be baked (as before described) into the muffle. Pure anthracite coal is the best for this purpose, as it maintains a longer and stronger heat than coke. Bituminous coal is not good for this kind of work unless first converted into coke.

"It often occurs that the natural gums will change more or less after the teeth are inserted. In such cases a new impression should be taken from the mouth and a fusible die formed. The denture is then placed upon the die, and it will be seen at once where the change has taken place, then with the piece resting upon the die the artificial gum may be chipped off with a small hammer and chisel. The platinum plate, being soft, can be refitted to the die very accurately with a burnisher, hammer, and small driver made for the purpose. A new coat of body is then applied where the plate has been refitted, and then baked, cooled, enameled, and baked again—still observing the same directions as detailed in the management of new pieces.

"If a tooth gets broken (a mishap which seldom occurs by use in the mouth), it can be replaced with another, by grinding out the remaining portion of the broken tooth, and the gum which covers the fang, and then fitting a new one in the place. This tooth need not be soldered to the inside rim; it is sufficient to grind a small notch or groove in the enamel which covers the lingual side of the rim for the pin of the tooth to fit into. The pin resting in the groove is covered with the body, at the same time it is applied around the base of the tooth, and when this body is baked the tooth will become firmly fastened in place of the broken one. Any number of teeth that may be required can be replaced in this way. If it is desired to change the position of one or more teeth, or to make them longer, this can also be done as described above, with this additional precaution, which is simply to press softened wax upon the inside of the teeth and palatal arch of the denture before the others are re- moved,—this wax will serve as a guide or index as to the relative change to be made, and also to sustain the teeth in place while they are being fitted as desired to the denture. The wax soon becomes hard and is readily removed as each successive tooth is ground and adjusted in its proper place.

" When the teeth are thus fitted with each pin accurately pressed into the groove prepared for it, and the wax being placed upon the inside to support the teeth in proper position,—body is filled in around the base of the new ones which are carved, trimmed and brushed, so as to have the crowns of the teeth clean and properly defined. The wax is then carefully removed from the piece, and more body is filled in around the teeth upon the inside,—filling up the grooves over the pins, and then carving, trimming, &c., as before, to give it the desired form. This done, if the teeth are set a little apart, and it is desired to keep them in that position, take a small piece of asbestos and gently press it in between the teeth at the cutting edges; this will prevent them from being drawn together when the body is being baked. The piece is now ready for the furnace, but it should not be baked hard enough to gloss the newly applied body; it should have more the appearance of Parian marble.

" This being done, it is then withdrawn from the furnace and transferred to a cooling muffle as before described. When sufficiently cool the gum enamel is applied and baked with a sharp heat until it becomes smooth and glossy. To prevent the old gum from bleaching or becoming lighter coloured in consequence of repeated bakings, a very thin coating of fresh gum enamel should be lightly brushed over the entire enameled surface of the piece. The enamel thus applied should be mixed with water, quite thin, so as to flow evenly over the surface, when applied with a camel's-hair brush. This should be done before the last baking, that the whole may be fused at the same time. Experience and judgment are essential requisites in order to produce good practical results. For example, if the carving of the body is not properly done, the form and shading of the gum and roof will not appear natural when the work is finished; if the gum enamel is put on too thick it will produce a dark red colour; if not thick enough it will be too light; if fused too hard it will be liable to craze or crack; if not hard enough it will be rough and granular; if the piece becomes gassed in baking it will be porous and of a bluish colour. Again, the teeth of different persons vary as much as any features of the face, and present as great a variety of expressions. Therefore, in the construction of artificial dentures, the dentist should select and arrange the teeth with special reference to each individual case. The length, size, form, shade, and position of the teeth should be varied to meet all the different physiognomical requirements that occur in dental practice.

" This system also combines with great advantage the restoration of the face in cases where the muscles have become sunken or fallen in from the loss of the teeth and consequent absorption of the alveolar processes. Here, again, the artistic skill of the dentist is brought into requisition. He should study the face of his patient as an artist studies his picture, for he displays his genius not upon canvas, but upon the living features of the face; and of how much more importance is the living picture, that reflects even the emotions of the heart, than the lifeless form upon canvas. He should know the origin and insertion of every muscle of which the face is formed, and what ones he is to raise, otherwise he will be liable to produce distortion instead of restoration. This improvement consists of prominences made upon the denture of such form and size as to bring out each muscle or sunken portion of the face to its original fulness; and when these are rightly formed they are not detected by the closest observer. There are four points of the face (of many persons) which the mere insertion of the teeth does not restore, viz., one upon each side beneath the malar or cheek bone, and also a point upon each side of the base of the nose, in a line toward the front portion of the malar bone.

" The extent of this falling-in varies in different persons, according to their temperaments. If the lymphatic temperament predominates, the change will be slight. If nervous or sanguine, it may be very great. The muscles situated upon the side of the face, and which rest upon the molar or back teeth, are the zygomaticus major, masseter, and buccinator. The loss of the above teeth causes these muscles to fall in. The principal mnscles which form the front portion of the face and lips are the zygomaticus minor, levator labii superioris alaeque nasi, and orbicularis oris.

" These rest upon the front, eye, and bicuspid teeth, which, when lost, allow the muscles to sink in, thereby changing the form and expression of the mouth.

" The insertion of the front teeth will in a great measure bring out the lips, but there are two muscles in the front portion of the face which cannot, in many cases, be thus restored to their original position; one is the zygomaticus minor, which arises from the front part of the malar bone, and is inserted into the upper lip above the angle of the mouth; the other is the levator muscle, which arises from the nasal process and from the edge of the orbit above the infra orbitar foramen. It is inserted into the ala nasi or wing of the nose and upper lip.

" The prominences before mentioned applied to these four points of the face, beneath the muscles just described, bring out that narrowness and sunken expression about the upper lip and cheeks to the same breadth and fulness which they formerly displayed. If skill and judgment have presided over all parts of the operation, the result will be highly pleasing, and of practical utility."

SECTION VIII

PIVOT TEETH

THE simplest arrangement for fixing a single tooth in the mouth, is by means of a pivot attached to the artificial tooth, and entering the canal of the pulp cavity of the natural tooth which has been already enlarged to receive it.

The cases most suitable for pivoting, are those in which the central incisors or canines of the upper jaw, have been fractured by accident, and have not decayed gradually away, leaving a soft broken down root in the gum. If the latter condition prevail, then the stump must be extracted, and not have an artificial crown pivoted on. Care and discretion must also be used not to treat patients who are of an inflammatory tendency, for they seldom do well, and on several occasions serious results have followed the apparently trifling operation of pivoting.

In the case also of the crown of the natural tooth having been lost from fracture, time must be allowed for the periostal inflammation to subside, before attempting to affix a new crown.

It seems hardly necessary to point out that if there be any evidence of alveolar abscess in the neighbourhood of the fang, there again this operation is inadmissible ; in fact, to put the matter in the most concise yet clear form, the stump must be perfectly healthy in every respect. If the stump is not fractured even with the line of the gum, or the decay of the crown has not entirely destroyed the tooth substance up to the neck, it will be necessary to remove by means of the tooth saw, and excising forceps, the portions projecting beyond the gum line. If but a small portion is remaining use the forceps alone, as the sensation of the saw is almost unendurable to many patients. When it is used, however, a cut must be commenced at the neck of the tooth on either the mesial or distal surface, and carried on towards the pulp cavity, following as nearly as possible the curvilinear margin of the gum. Before the pulp cavity is reached on the one side the saw must be removed and applied in the same manner to the opposite side ; we then have the crown supported by a ridge of bony tissue in the centre, running from before backwards. This can be now readily divided with the excising forceps.

Care must be taken not to saw into the pulp on account of the pain, but it is well to get nearly into the pulp-cavity, as it renders excision much easier. The form of saw and forceps used for this operation are shown in the annexed engraving.

FIG. 68.

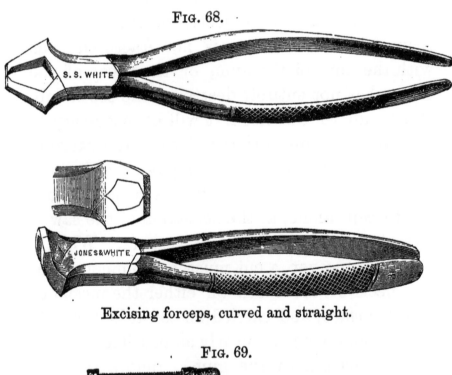

Excising forceps, curved and straight.

FIG. 69.

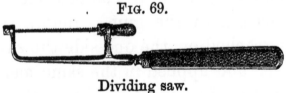

Dividing saw.

Under ordinary circumstances, the nerve will now be exposed to view; if possible pass a nerve extractor, Fig 70, into the cavity, and withdraw the pulp, or use an ordinary FIG. 70. untempered brooch, passing this up and then twisting sharply round so as to destroy the connection of the nerve filament. It may then be removed easily with the barbed nerve extractor, if it should not come out on the brooch. It is never wise, and seldom safe, to use arsenic for the destruction of the nerve where pivoting is to be performed. It is much better if there is likely to be much trouble on account of the nervousness of the patient, to destroy the nerve, before cutting down the stump, by repeated applications of Pepsina porci and dilute hydrochloric acid, as recommended in my notes on 'Dental Pathology.'

The pulp-cavity being now clear must be enlarged for the reception of the pivot. This can be done with one or other of the instruments shown in Fig. 71, gradually increasing the size until the requisite diameter has been obtained. In young subjects, care must be taken not to drill through the pulp cavity in the apex of the tooth, lest you pass into the investing membrane of the fang. It is well at this stage to file down the rough edges of the

stump, so as to present a perfectly smooth surface, convex from back to front and concave
from side to side, on which the crown of the
pivot tooth may be fitted. The most convenient
way of fitting the crown to the fang is to make
a temporary wooden or wire pivot, that will

FIG. 71.

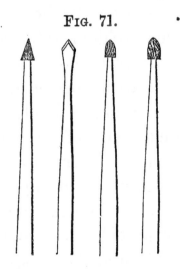

pass easily in and out of the fang, with half an
inch of the point projecting into the mouth. A
wax impression may now be taken of the stump
and adjacent teeth. When this is removed
from the mouth the wooden pivot will be seen
standing in the wax. On the model being cast
from this the temporary pivot will occupy the
same relative position as when in the mouth,
and by removing it we have the fang cavity
reproduced also, which will act as a guide for
the direction of the pivot.

The choice of the tooth is a most important thing, of greater moment for pivot cases than for any other, since they generally are isolated, and if not matched perfectly for shape and colour produce a most unsatisfactory result by the side of the natural teeth. One of three varieties may be used. Either a pivot tooth proper, Fig. 72, a tube tooth fitted with a pivot, Fig. 73 ; or a flat tooth with a gold back and a gold or platina pivot soldered on, Fig. 74.

FIG. 72.   FIG. 73.   FIG. 74.

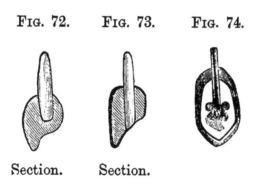

Section.   Section.

The advantage of the tooth made expressly for pivoting, is the perfect resemblance to the natural crown, and from the fact that the tube does not pass right through, enabling the operator to use compressed hickory wood as a pivot pin.

The advantage of a tube tooth is its greater strength, being used with a metal pin, and having a platina tube down the centre, which the first description of tooth has not, whilst its great disadvantage is that the pinhole is rarely in precisely the right place, being generally too near the face of the tooth.

The benefit of using a flat tooth is especially seen in a close bite, where there is little room for either a pivot or tube tooth, or when, from the abnormal position of the pulp-cavity, an ordinary tooth is not available.   In these cases the pin can be arranged in almost any position that can possibly be required, since there is ample room for adjustment by reason of the thinness of the tooth.   The only objection to its use is the rough surface presented in the mouth, and its relative fragility.

The model when obtained had better be dipped or varnished, or a little resin and wax run over it before fitting the tooth, in order to prevent wearing away of the surface of the stump as shown in the plaster.

The tooth must be ground at the lathe with a corundum wheel, Fig. 75, and then finely fitted by colouring the model over the stump with vermilion and oil, and noting the points of contact when the tooth is put on the stump; these will be indicated by the colour adhering, and must be ground away till all the surface of the tooth is in perfect contact with the stump.

Care must be taken to adjust the tooth and pivot together in fitting, so that they may not occupy a malposition when fixed in the mouth.

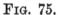

Fig. 75.

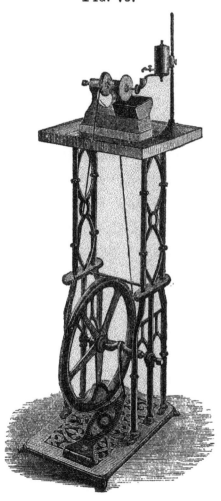

Some dental surgeons prefer fitting the tooth to the stump direct in the patient's mouth, colouring the stump for fine fitting.

This process is, however, tedious to both patient and operator, as well as being somewhat disagreeable to the former. The tooth being fitted, the pivot, if of wood, must be made so as to pass firmly but not tightly into the pulp-canal, and somewhat tightly into the tube of the pivot tooth ; it will not do, however to apply too much force in introducing either, lest you should crack the tooth or give pain in the stump when the wood has begun to swell from the moisture. Previous to finally fixing the pivot, syringe the pulp-cavity with a weak solution of carbolic acid and water, then plug the extremity of the nerve canal either with gold or cotton wool soaked in creasote, or osteo-plastic carefully applied, so as to seal up the extreme opening of the canal.

The wooden pivot may be wrapped round with one or two layers of gold foil, thus protecting both the pivot and the walls of the fang from the action of the secretions of the mouth.

No greater pressure than can be applied with the thumb and finger should be required for adjusting a wood pivot, as the swelling that takes place will quickly render it quite firm.

Wooden pivots may be strengthened if desired by drilling carefully down the centre after fitting, and passing a gold or platina wire through.

If a metal pivot is used then it must be fastened into the artificial crown with powdered sulphur placed over the opening of the tube in the tooth, and melted carefully over a spirit lamp. The pin at this part having been previously roughened will be held quite secure by this method. For adjustment to the dental canal, the extremity of the pin may be roughened or slightly barbed, and then fitted in with floss silk wound round, and coated with mastic, or the cavity may be filled with osteo-plastic, and the pivot introduced while the stopping is in a soft state. The attachment of the pin to a flat tooth I shall treat of further on.

It is impossible to enumerate in a work of the present nature all the ingenious contrivances that have been introduced for the fixing of pivot teeth. Each plan has some special merit of its own, but the methods that I have described are those most widely in use, and are open to the fewest practical objections.

SECTION IX

CHOOSING AND ADJUSTING MINERAL TEETH

ABOVE all other departments of the Dental Surgeon's work, the choosing and adjusting of mineral teeth gives the fullest opportunity for the display of sound judgment and artistic feeling.

In all reproductions nature must be imitated, but not servilely copied. Utility must be borne in mind, but not at the sacrifice of appearance and beauty, still less must we forget the special services which the teeth perform in the human economy. Every condition requisite may be fulfilled, by the exercise of those faculties to which I have already alluded.

For partial cases it is essential, above all things, that the shape and texture of the teeth, should be reproduced in the artificial substitutes, as well as the mere colour and shade. The first are the marks of individuality, the last merely a matter of complexion, and are in the natural organ subject to variation.

Beware how you reproduce in the mouth deformities, that have resulted from the malformation, or arrangement of the teeth. Though your work be true to nature, you will but rarely find a patient sufficiently educated up to your stand-point, to appreciate your skill in this respect. If irregularities of the natural organs are imitated in the artificial teeth, it must be done with great care and discretion, as the same amount of displacement —say of the laterals—will not be tolerated in the reproduction, that was present in the original arrangement.

In choosing teeth for partial cases there is, of course, the guidance given as to shape and shade by the remaining teeth, but where the gums are edentulous, and you have not had the opportunity of seeing any of the patient's natural teeth, you must be guided in your choice, by the size and shape of the gums, and then by the complexion and characteristics of your patient. As a broad rule, it may be laid down that it is wiser to use artificial teeth, of a somewhat smaller size than the natural ones. When an entire set is fitted in, the result is more pleasing by following this plan than if large teeth were used, however natural they may be in actual dimensions.

Leaving these general observations, we will now pass on to the more special consideration of—

Adjusting and fixing teeth to partial cases. —However carefully the teeth may have been chosen, they will scarcely fit into their respective places, without some amount of grinding with the corundum wheel at the lathe. If the stumps are remaining, or there be but slight absorption, then the tooth must be fitted on the gum at its anterior and lateral borders, but the remaining portion may rest on the plate. If an artificial tooth has to be fitted on a stump care must be taken to have the stump filed down level with the gum. On the plaster model, this portion should be covered with resin and wax in solution, (if the model has not been dipped) so that it may not be 'worn away, with the fitting of the tooth to its surface. Should the model become at all injured on the surface, the artificial tooth will ride on the stump in the mouth, and if it does not do this, the mineral tooth will soon be broken, from the extra pressure that is brought to bear upon it.

When, however, the teeth are to rest upon the gum only, the stumps having been removed, it is advisable to scrape the plaster model away slightly, so that the contact may be perfect between the artificial teeth and the gums, when the plate is fitted into the mouth.

As to the adjustment of teeth to awkward bites or articulations, it is difficult to give directions that will be of much service in practice. It will be necessary to sacrifice utility for appearance in the arrangement of the teeth for partial cases, situated in the anterior portion of the mouth; but with cases for the masticatory region, I should unreservedly reverse this order, and sacrifice appearance for usefulness. On both points, it is well to make up your own mind firmly, and then abide by it; once submit to the dictates or suggestions of your patient, and your peace of mind and conscience are gone; it is better to lose a patient than to submit to the discomfort that will inevitably ensue if you follow their instructions or fulfil their desires (contrary to your own judgment).

It is sometimes desirable to raise the bite slightly (that is, not allow the patient to close the mouth so much as formerly); this must be done very carefully and to a very slight extent, or great discomfort will be caused, and by destroying the perfect articulation injury will be done to any teeth still standing in the mouth. When, however, the teeth posterior to the incisors of the upper and lower jaws are absent, and the front teeth are being worn away, and the upper incisors protruded by the pressure brought to bear upon them, great benefit will follow raising the bite to such an extent at the back of the mouth with the artificial denture, as to relieve the undue pressure that has been exercised in front.

After the teeth are fitted to the model and attached to the plate by means of resin and wax, they must be tried in the mouth, and any alteration that is necessary, made at once, as after they are soldered on it will be difficult to readjust them.

Investing in plaster and sand or asbestos,— presuming that the teeth are for plate—some use both the latter substances, adding only sufficient plaster, to produce cohesion of the other materials—they must be mixed to a tolerably stiff paste, and placed on a smooth surface, with a square of paper underneath so as to allow of easy removal; the plate with the teeth attached is then pressed gently down, so that all the lower surface is well supported, and the teeth surrounded on their labial surface, with the plaster and sand, so that when trimmed up, a thickness of nearly half an inch is left around them.

As soon as the plaster and sand is sufficiently hard to bear handling, the resin and
wax must be cleansed away thoroughly, and
the backs fitted to the teeth and plate. A
plan practised in America is to remove the
teeth from the investing material carefully, and
fit the backs on. The more general practice
in England is to fit the backings of the teeth
after fitting them on to the plate, but before
investing in plaster, and the latter is, I think,
a better method; the backing in either case
must be somewhat thinner than the metal used
for the plate, and should be stiffened, by the
addition of platinum as an alloy.

The holes for the pins of the teeth, may be
either drilled, punched out, or perforated with
a pair of pliers of the form shown in the accompanying cut, Fig. 76.

FIG. 76.

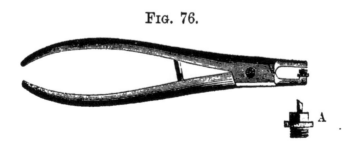

These nippers are so arranged that the
cutting-pins can be renewed as often as necessary. This is accomplished by unscrewing the

movable socket A, and dropping in the pin from the back. The pins are flattened at the opposite end, to prevent them turning round or falling through, and when the socket A is screwed home in the head of the nippers the pin is secure.

The plate being fitted to the back of the tooth, ·the rivets are then split with a scorper and spread outwards; as soon as all the backings are fitted satisfactorily, the joints must be strengthened by means of fine gold wire cut off to the width of the tooth, and bent so as to fit accurately at the base of the backing, thus increasing the strength and giving stiffness and solidity to the piece. Where the bite requires it metal boxes may be made and attached to the backs, but for such a case it will be better as a rule to use a tooth that of itself gives a masticating surface. When these things are done, the pins being thoroughly cleansed, must be coated with borax and water, wherever it is necessary for the solder to flow. The borax can be prepared by rubbing on a piece of slate or porcelain with water, till the fluid is of a creamy consistence.

The solder must be carefully placed in every position where it will be required, so as to avoid having to use more after the piece is made hot;

everything being arranged in a satisfactory manner the piece is placed in the hand furnace and gradually warmed up, then the top of the furnace may be removed, and the heat applied with the blowpipe till the mass is of a bright red colour; the well-directed flame of the blowpipe will by this time cause the solder to flow in every direction required; or instead of this plan the piece invested in the plaster may be taken out of the furnace when sufficiently hot, and placed on a slab of charcoal (surrounded with plaster of Paris), and the heat then raised by the aid of the blowpipe.

The first plan is, however, the best, unless it be a very small case that requires soldering.

For full sets of teeth, the same rules and modes of procedure apply as for a partial set; it is necessary, however, to adopt some plan to prevent the plaster and sand breaking, when the denture is being warmed up in the furnace, or during the time of soldering.

Some pass two or three pieces of iron or copper binding wire round the teeth, before investing in plaster and sand, others use a strip of copper, somewhat in the shape of the outline of the gum, thus affording a support to the outer surface of the plaster. A plan that I deem better still, however, is to obtain a shallow saucer, with perpendicular sides, made of fire-clay or plumbago, and after filling this with plaster and asbestos or sand, sink the denture in it and thus use the saucer at once as a support, and a means of retaining the heat, after it is taken from the furnace for soldering.

As soon as the soldering is completed, remove the piece from the furnace, and place it on cold charcoal or pumice stone to cool down.

Some recommend cooling down at once, by pouring boiling water, over the plaster and sand, no risk being run of cracking the teeth ; but it is better to wait a little longer, and let the plaster cool of itself.

After removing the plaster and sand, or asbestos, as the case may be, the plate should be thoroughly washed in water, and then boiled in a solution of sulphuric acid (one part acid, two parts water) so as to destroy the borax, that has become fused and attached to the gold. Scorpers of the form shown for finishing up vulcanite work, can now be used to remove any projecting portions of solder or wire strengthening that has been applied, or these may be cut down at the lathe with a fine corundum wheel and plenty of water. The entire surface must be then rendered smooth by means of Ayrstone and water and a stick and pumice powder, then polished at the lathe, first with pumice powder and a hard brush, then with whiting and a softer brush, and, finally, with rouge and a softer brush still, commencing this last stage with the brush wet, and working at it till the brush becomes dry. For those spaces where a brush cannot be applied, two or three threads, fixed at one end to the work bench, may be passed through or between the space to be polished, and the plates passed up and down these threads (which should be loaded with a little of the polishing material) until a smooth and polished surface is obtained. Strips of tape and cord may also be used for the same purpose, using a different size according to necessity. After this the plate must be thoroughly cleaned with hot soda and water, and dried in a bag filled with box-wood dust. The case is now ready for fitting in the mouth.

Fitting tube teeth to a full set.—These should first be roughly fitted down to the plate, and the gum as well, if they are to overlap the edge of the plate, each tooth as it is fitted in this way being attached to the plate by means of cement, such as I have recommended for flat teeth, and in this way the entire denture must be mounted up so as to assume the form re-

quired in the finished set, allowing just sufficient excess of tooth surface for fine fitting.
As soon as they are all suitably arranged, a
finely pointed broach must be passed down each
tube very carefully and rotated, so as to leave
a mark over the plate, or, instead of this, a
piece of straight steel wire with a flat extremity
may be dipped in a mixture of vermilion and
oil, and then lightly dropped down the tube of
the tooth, thus marking with the point the
position for the pin. Or still another plan may
be adopted ; imbed the front of the teeth and
model in plaster up to the level of the tops of
the teeth (after soaping their surfaces) ; then
fill in the palatine surface also with plaster ;
this will keep the teeth in position, and as soon
as it is set, the holes in the plate may be made
by means of an Archimedean drill passing down
the tubes of the teeth ; in this way the direction
of the tube is continued into the perforation of
the plate, and the pin can be applied and soldered in, so as to avoid the necessity of bending
afterwards. Before the pins canbe fitted to
the plate the plaster overcastings must of
course be removed with the teeth. When the
pins are all in good position the teeth may be
fine fitted, by means of the vermilion and oil
and a small-grained corundum wheel.

Tube teeth are attached to the pins and plate, by means of sulphur ground to a coarse powder. The plate with teeth on, is made hot over a spirit lamp and the sulphur then applied; as it melts with the heat it runs down the tubes of the teeth, and on hardening retains them quite firmly in position. After this the ends of the pins which project may be ground down at the lathe, so as to be flush with the surface of the teeth.

SECTION X

THE VULCANITE BASE

In a work that is intended to be thoroughly practical in its nature, it is neither wise nor necessary, to go into the history of the invention of every substance treated of. On this account I shall make no reference to the successive patents, trials, disputes, and works that have been published upon the vulcanite base, but shall confine myself to its composition, properties, and uses.

The toughest and strongest rubber in every way is that which is sold as uncoloured or brown rubber. It contains the largest proportion of the natural gum, mixed with one of the various forms of sulphur, and is not deteriorated by the introduction of any colouring matter. From this rubber all the other varieties may be said to be built up.

The manufacture of the different rubbers

used, is a secret kept very securely by the makers. From the experiments, however, of Professor Wildman (of Philadelphia) contained in his ' Instructions in Vulcanite,' we are able to form a very fair judgment as to the composition and mode of treating this valuable natural product.

" Caoutchouc may be mixed with sulphur, and the colouring matter, by being passed repeatedly between steam-heated rollers ; or the caoutchouc may be first reduced to a pulpy or gelatinous state by some one of its solvents, and the sulphur and colouring matter then mixed with it ; in either case the sulphur and colouring should be ground extremely fine, and then the whole ingredients thoroughly incorporated together to ensure a satisfactory result.

" For experimental purposes the latter method of mixing can be readily practised by any one. Of the solvents, ether deprived of its alcohol, chloroform and bisulphide of carbon are objectionable on account of their expense, and also the operator being compelled to inhale their vapour during the manipulation. Coal naphtha, or benzine, are preferable on this account ; they readily reduce the caoutchouc to the proper consistency ; but after having been mixed, and the solvent evaporated, the rubber is non-adhesive, and does not pack well. Oil of turpentine leaves the rubber somewhat adhesive, and in a good condition to pack. Therefore I have found it a better plan to soften the caoutchouc in oil of turpentine, or in equal parts of cold naptha, or benzine, and oil of turpentine.

"In reducing caoutchouc to a gelatinous condition, it requires a large quantity of the solvent in proportion to the gum. This is remedied by introducing into the solvent from five to fifty per cent. of alcohol; in this case the caoutchouc becomes gelatinous, but does diffuse itself through the solvent, thereby leaving much of it after the softened caoutchouc is removed, for future use.

"I generally levigate the colouring matter and sulphur in spirits of turpentine, first reducing the colouring matter very fine, then adding the sulphur, and also reducing it very fine, then add a little of the pulpy caoutchouc, mix thoroughly, and proceed in this manner until the whole is incorporated into a perfectly homogeneous mass. When the colouring matter is ground in linseed oil, the caoutchouc may be softened in naphtha, or benzine, and it will pack well, as the oil renders it adhesive; but I am inclined to believe that oil, even in a small quantity, injures the hardness and polish of the rubber.

" After the materials are well mixed the mass should be spread on a glass plate with a spatula, and allowed to remain until the solvent has been evaporated.

" The apparatus used in making the following mixtures were a muller and glass plate to grind the colours and sulphur, a spatula, broad-mouth bottles, in which to gelatinize the caoutchouc, and window glass, upon which to spread it when mixed. The caoutchouc was the best Para, and the time and temperature in vulcanizing was the same as that for the American Hard Rubber Company's red rubber.

" *To test the Combination of Caoutchouc and Sulphur alone :*

    1. Caoutchouc   48
        Sulphur   24

This gave a dark brown rubber, varying shade in different mixtures ; it was strong, compact, and tough, and received a fine polish. This colour may be toned down to a dark oak by bleaching in alcohol.

" 2· This experiment was performed with caoutchouc which had not been smoked ; this gum was translucent and nearly colourless, having merely a light straw tint. The proportions were the same as for 1.

" *Result.*—Colour and properties the same as the above, showing that the natural colour of hard rubber composed of simply caoutchouc and sulphur is a dark brown.

" *To test the Colouring Properties of Red Oxide of Iron.*—The following formula gave the best results of the many tried :

```
 ··    3.  Caoutchouc    .    .    .    .    48
           Sulphur  .    .    .    .    .    24
           Red oxide of iron (rouge).    .    36
```

" *Result.*—Texture good ; colour in different mixtures varied from almost black to black red ; the colour was more on the red when the rouge was ground in oil than when in spirits of turpentine ; after exposure in alcohol to the rays of the sun, the red was better developed, but even then it was much darker than the Company's red rubber. The sulphur decomposed the oxide of iron, forming a dark sulphide, thereby destroying its colouring effect.

" *Vermilion for producing a Red.*—Numerous experiments were tried to ascertain the quantity of vermilion necessary to overcome the natural brown and produce a red colour ; the following mixture may be set down as the lowest :

4. Caoutchouc	.	.	.	.	48
Sulphur	.	.	.	.	24
Vermilion	.	.	.	.	36

"Some mixtures made according to this formula were darker and some lighter, owing to the different varieties of vermilion used. The shade was made much lighter by bleaching in alcohol. To bring it to a bright red when vulcanized would require much more vermilion, perhaps equal proportions of caoutchouc and vermilion. This formula produced a good, strong, compact rubber. If not identical in composition with the Company's red, it so closely resembles it in texture, strength, and appearance, and in every particular it must very nearly approximate thereto.

"*To produce a Yellow.*—The colouring effect of chrome yellow was tested; it gave a slate colour, the chromate of lead being decomposed, setting free the chromic acid, and forming a sulphide of lead, stone ochre, and Naples yellow and the common orpiment of commerce, were tried with no better results. Pure orpiment or king's yellow gave, when bleached, a lemon yellow, when mixed as follows :

5. Caoutchouc	.	.	.	.	48
Sulphur	.	.	.	.	24
King's yellow	.	.	.	.	36

" Although the colour produced by this substance was much more satisfactory than any of the preceding, its use is objectionable, because the texture of the rubber was not good, and the king's yellow being sulphide of arsenic is very poisonous.

" The following formula gives a good reliable yellow, viz. :

6.	Caoutchouc	48
	Sulphur	24
	Sulphide of cadmium . .	36

" This requires bleaching to develope the colour fully ; it is then much better than that produced by orpiment, is more on the orange, the texture of the rubber is good, and its use is not objectionable.

" *For a Lighter Yellow—*

7.	Caoutchouc	48
	Sulphur	36
	Sulph. ed.	36
	White ox. zinc	12

" The white oxide of zinc toned down the deep yellow to more of a lemon colour, similar to that produced by the orpiment, at the same time the rubber was of good texture.

" Experiments to produce a pink and a flesh-colour so far have not been successful in producing the desired results, yet some of them are worthy of note.

8.	Caoutchouc	. . . .	48
	Sulphur	. . . . .	24
	White ox. zinc .	. . .	30
	Vermilion	. . . .	10

" When bleached, gave a dark pink, the colour not so good as the English ; texture close ; not so strong as the brown or red.

" *Variation of the above.*

9.	Caoutchouc	. . . .	48
	Sulphur	. . . . .	24
	White ox. zinc .	. . .	36
	Vermilion	. . . .	10

" Vulcanized brown, after bleaching ; it was a shade lighter than the preceding.

" The mixture of

10.	Caoutchouc	. . . .	48
	Sulphur	. . . . .	24
	White ox. zinc .	. . .	48
	E. vermilion	. . . .	10
	Sulphide of cadmium	. .	6

after bleaching, produced a buff.

" *Variation of above.*

11.	Caoutchouc	. . . .	48
	Sulphur	. . . . .	24
	White ox. zinc .	. . .	96
	Vermilion	. . . .	5
	Sulphide of cadmium	. .	3

This produced a lighter shade—a light buff.

" To ascertain the effect of white oxide of zinc upon the natural brown of vulcanized rubber, numerous mixtures were made. The best Lehigh white oxide was used.

12.	Caoutchouc	48
	Sulphur	24
	White ox. zinc	36

" This produced a drab after bleaching—texture good.

13.	Caoutchouc	48
	Sulphur	24
	White oxide of zinc . . .	48

"When bleached gave a light drab of good texture, and in appearance approximates very near to that of the American Hard Rubber Company's white.

14.	Caoutchouc	48
	Sulphur	24
	White oxide of zinc . . .	96

" This after bleaching gave a grayish white. These three preceding mixtures were repeated by varying the proportion of sulphur, substituting thirty-six for twenty-four; the object of this was to give the rubber additional hardness; this change of proportions had the desired effect, but at the same time the colour was impaired. All of these mixtures vulcanize a brownish colour, and require to be bleached by the rays of the sun in alcohol for their development.

" *To produce a Black* Rubber.

15.	Caoutchouc	.	.	.	.	48
	Sulphur .	.	.	.	.	24
	Ivory black, or drop black			.		24

" This mixture gave a good black.

16.	Caoutchouc	.	.	.	.	48
	Sulphur .	.	.	.	.	24
	Ivory, or drop black			.	.	48

" This produced an excellent *jet black*, the rubber was hard and of good texture.

" The drop black which is in lumps containing gum I have uniformly found to produce a porous rubber, whilst the article under the same name found in commerce, free from gum, gave good results.

" By taking several of these different mixtures (such as the taste of the operator may dictate), and cutting them into shreds, then incorporating them together, and again cutting the mass into small pieces suitable for packing, a very pretty mottled rubber may be made suitable for hurdles, &c.

" After being vulcanized and polished, it must be bleached in alcohol to fully develope

the colours, although some of the mixtures
present a pleasing appearance without the
bleaching process.

" In finishing mottled rubber, owing to the
several coloured mixtures having a different
degree of hardness, after the file, prepare for
the polishing process by obliterating the file
marks with a flat piece of Scotch stone.

" The introduction of shellac was tried in one
experiment, viz. :

Caoutchouc	48
Sulphur	24
Vermilion	40
Shellac	12

" The addition of shellac did appear to improve the compound in appearance or texture.

" I have now presented the most interesting
of the successful results of my expériments in
compounding mixtures for making hard rubber,
and would now call the attention of those who
desire to pursue this subject experimentally,
that to colour rubber three points are essential : First, the colour must remain unchanged
at the heat required for vulcanization. Second,
it must withstand the action of sulphur at this
tempèrature ; and third, sufficient quantity
must be added to the mixture to overpower the
natural brown of vulcanized rubber, before its

shade can be developed. This fact shows us that all highly coloured rubbers, or where the brown is widely departed from, must be weakened by their being loaded with so much colour or foreign matter; in proof of this I have found no other mixture possessing strength and toughness equal to that made of simply caoutchouc and sulphur.

" The following table gives, very nearly, the percentage of caoutchouc contained in several of the preceding formula. Also that of Ash and Sons' Pink No. 1, their S. P., their white, and the white made by the American Hard Rubber Company. The percentage given by these latter is based upon calculation.

" From the results of the preceding experiments it is evident we may substitute Ash and Sons' black and the American Hard Rubber Company's brown for the 1 brown in the table. Also the English deep red and the American Hard Rubber Company's red for 4, the red in the table.

		Caoutchouc.	Sulphur.	Vermilion.			Parts in
1.	Brown	66⅔	33⅓				100
4.	Red	44	22	33			99
6.	Yellow	44	22			Sulph. Cad. 33	99
8.	Pink	43⅔	21⅓	9		Ox. Zn. 27	100
11.	Buff	35·4	17·2×	7·3	4·4	Sulph. Cad. 35·4	100

	Caoutchouc.	Sulphur.	Vermilion.	Ox. Zn.	Parts in
14. Drab . . .	44	. 22	. .	. 33	. 99
15. Lighter Drab .	40	. 20	. .	. 40	.
16. Grayish White .	28·5	. 14·3	. .	. 57·1+	100
				Black.	
17. Black . . .	50	. 25	. .	. 25	. 100
18. Jet . . .	40	. 20	. .	. 40	. 100
				White earthy matter.	
Ash & Sons' Pink, No. 1	24	. 12	. 18 .	. 48	. 102
				Ox. Zn.	
,, ,, S. P .	35·6	. 17·3	.26·6.	. 20	. 100
,, ,, White .	32⅔	. 16⅓	. .	. 51	. 100
Am. H. R. Co.'s White	32⅔	. 16⅓	. .	. 51	. 100

" The calculation for the component parts of Ash and Sons' Pink Rubber is based upon the method given in the patent for making pink rubber for dental uses, the quantity of fixed matter it is found to contain, and taking formula 4 as the composition of red rubber. It will be found, upon examination of this data, that, if there is any error in the quantity of caoutchouc given to the pink, it is in its favour. A glance at the table will at once show its and other light rubbers' inferiority to either brown or red for dental purposes.

" The calculation of the percentage of Ash and Sons' S. P. is based upon the quantity of fixed matter found in it, and that fixed matter having been mixed a red rubber compound as in formula 4. This is evidently superior to the pink, but inferior either to the red or brown.

" Caoutchouc being the *cement* which binds the whole together, if any compound should contain but a small proportion of it, and if any substance prejudicial to the system should enter into its composition (and in the patent referred to for making pink rubber, such substances are recommended), its weakness of texture from the want of sufficient adhesion of its particles would render it liable to produce injurious effects by its susceptibility to abrasion in the mouth."

Some very interesting experiments were also made by Prof. Wildman to ascertain, by the application of heat, the amount of fixed matter contained in various specimens of rubber compounds. A condensed statement of the results obtained is exhibited in the following table :

	Per cent. of fixed matter.	
1. Specimens of Deep Pink . . .	60	
2. English Pink	48	White Clay.
3. Ash & Sons' Pale Pink, No. 1 .	48	,, ,,
4. ,, ,, Deep Pink, No. 1, X	47	Oxide of Zinc.
5. ,, ,, S. P.	20	,, ,,
6. ,, ,, Black . . .	4	Dark Ash.
7. ,, ,, White . . .	51	White Ox. Zic.
8. English Red	6	Dark Ash.
9. Dieffenbach's Red	16	,, ,,

11

					Per cent of fixed matter.
10. Am. H. R. Co.'s Red	.	.	.	.	Dark Ash.
11. " White	.	.	.	51	White Ox. Zic.
12. " Brown, near	.	.	4	Dark Ash.
13. My own Brown (C 2, S 1) near	.	.	3	" "
14. " Red (C 48, S. 24, V. 36)	.	2	" "

The author observes: " These experiments show us that pink and light rubbers for dental purposes are heavily loaded with such foreign matter as white clay and oxide of zinc, and some to the extent of fifty-one per cent. of their weight. Ash and Sons' S. P. is decidedly the best of his light rubbers, containing only twenty per cent. of fixed matter.

" Again, Ash and Sons' black (brown), the American Hard Rubber Company's brown, and my own brown, give results, respectively four, near four, and near three per cent. of fixed matter. My own, I know, was made of pure caoutchouc and of sulphur; hence from the residues of the two former so nearly approximating thereto, and also from their similarity of texture and appearance after being vulcanized, we must arrive at the conclusion they are of the same composition, and are therefore good and reliable brown rubbers.

" When we examine the results of the experiments upon the English deep red, that made by the American Hard Rubber Company, and my own red, we find the fixed matter to be six, five, and two per cent. respectively. My own red was made of pure Para caoutchouc, vermilion, and sulphur. The small disparity of fixed matter found in these rubbers may have arisen from the different state of purity of the caoutchouc used in compounding them.

"It is evident that the specimens of English Red and of the American Hard Rubber Company's red were not loaded with earthy matter or oxides of zinc or lead, for if they were, the clay would have given us a greater percentage of fixed matter. Oxide of zinc is fixed in the fire at a white heat, and if present would have produced a similar result. Oxide of lead would have shown itself by its reduction, and the greater weight of residue.

"The conclusion we would naturally arrive at from the results of these experiments is, that the American Hard Rubber Company's red, and the English deep red, are the best red rubbers offered for dental purposes."

The properties of vulcanite are extreme hardness and toughness when subjected to the action of super-heated steam for a variable time (according to composition); extreme softness and elasticity when composed with a special view to that result or when vulcanised in a pecnliar manner which I shall hereafter refer to, extreme lightness, the power of resisting most chemical agents, whilst it is not acted upon by any ordinary degree of heat, such, for instance, as the temperature of the mouth. Its chief advantage, however, is the facility with which it can be adapted to any form and receive a perfect and sharp impression from any hard counterpart into which it may be pressed.

With regard to the uses of vulcanite in dental surgery and mechanics, they are innumerable; in almost all cases where gold was formerly used exclusively, vulcanite can now be applied instead; whilst in place of bone work, vulcanite may be always employed with equal advantage, and very often with greater comfort to the patient.

This material has, however, been used more extensively for regulating plates (superseding gold and bone work) than for any other purpose in dental mechanics, since, from its peculiar properties and market value, greater facilities are offered to the operator for the frequent renewal of mechanical contrivances for regulating the teeth.

Under their several departments the various

forms and manners in which vulcanite is used will be treated of.

When vulcanite was first introduced numerous cases were reported of salivation being produced, owing to the presence of sulphuret of mercury as a colouring agent. Some of these were, doubtless, well and clearly marked; but it is not improbable that others were due to the prejudice with which the new base was received by a large number of those practising dentistry. There is no question that some of the earlier and carelessly prepared specimens of vulcanite did contain mischievous agents, but in the present day, rubber purchased of makers of good repute need give no occasion for alarm to the most scrupulous of practitioners.

In another part of the work will be found the time and temperature advised for cooking the various descriptions of rubber which are used; there are, however, certain general conditions that may be best discussed in the present section. Whenever practicable the flask should occupy a central position in the vulcanizer, and should not rest on metal, but pumice stone, so that heat may not be communicated by conduction to one part more than another. For all varieties of rubber the longer the time, and the more slowly the temperature is raised the better; thus, a piece will come out tougher and stronger in every way, by being vulcanized four hours at a low temperature, rather than an hour and a quarter at 315°, and with elastic rubber especially six or even eight hours are a great advantage.

The most obvious evil resulting from rapid vulcanizing is porosity of the rubber, and this is undoubtedly caused, as Professor Wildman points out, by the rapid evolution of sulphur-etted-hydrogen gas, and its confinement to the central portion of the block of rubber by the superficial hardening of the external layer only of the denture. This evolution of gas during vulcanizing is, in fact, proved to demonstration by the following experiment of the Professor :

" To ascertain if sulphuretted-hydrogen is given off during vulcanization, a bulb was blown at the end of a glass tube; this was filled with red rubber, the tube was then drawn out very small from immediately above the bulb, and curved so that the small part when the bulb was in the paraffin bath could be inserted into a vessel beside it.

" The bulb was then placed in a paraffin bath and the curved end of the tube inserted in a vessel containing a solution of acetate of lead.

The heat was raised to 320° F., and retained at that point for one hour and a quarter.

" The mean results of several experiments conducted in this manner were, that during the first thirty or forty minutes after the heat had attained to 320°, bubbles of sulphuretted-hydrogen came over at short intervals, and at the expiration of this time it was evolved in a continuous stream which continued for a few minutes, causing a copious precipitate of sulphide of lead. After this, until the expiration of the hour and a quarter, the gas was only given off sparingly at intervals. This experiment gives us ocular demonstration that this gas is evolved during vulcanization, and in large quantities, and conclusively shows that in thick pieces, especially, the heat should be slowly raised, and the rubber should be under strong pressure to ensure a successful result."

To construct a full upper set of teeth in the vulcanite base.—The impression of the mouth should always be taken in plaster of Paris, and the model cast so that its thinnest part may not be more than half an inch thick; this will prevent the trouble of cutting it down after the teeth are mounted ready for flasking, and admits of its being placed in the articulating frame up to the last moment, to make sure that no displacement has taken place. I must, for the moment, suppose that the model has been fitted up to an articulation in a bite frame, so that we may proceed to the mounting of the teeth. A plate of wax rolled out to the thickness of a sixteenth of an inch may be softened by the spirit lamp, or in warm water, and pressed carefully all over the upper surface of the model, that is, the palate and alveolar ridge; or thin gutta percha may be used, which is better when it has to be tried in the mouth (especially in hot weather). Another plan that I have adopted, and like very much, is to take some good white or pink blotting-paper, not too thick, warm it before the fire, or on a hot plate, then immerse in melted wax, letting the superfluous wax drip off, and allowing the wax to harden, then cut out patterns from this according to size and shape, and having softened the pattern before the fire, apply it in the same way as the wax plate or thin gutta percha. There are several advantages connected with this mode of action: you obtain a more equal thickness (by applying a number of layers as you require them); you do not by extra pressure reduce the substance where there are prominent ridges in the gums, as you may do with wax, or even gutta percha, and at the same time you have a tougher base to rely upon when trying the set in the patient's mouth.

Still another plan, more troublesome, but infinitely better in its results, is that known as "Stent's process;" it consists of mounting up the plate in a soft metal in thin sheets (about No. 6 gauge); they must be struck up with a zinc or tin model in lead, and may be composed of one or more layers of metal, but when finished they are very strong and neat, and the teeth may be fitted on to them with wax in the same way as when wax, gutta percha, or paper are used.

The plate, whatever the material used, being fitted to the model perfectly, must be trimmed up to the required size, as shown in accompanying drawing (Fig. 77). As a rule, it may

FIG. 77.

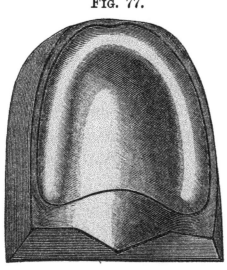

extend all round to the extent of the impression, except posteriorly, that is, if the patient has been allowed to nearly close the mouth when taking the impression; plaster of Paris gives the most accurate representations of all the delicate folds of membrane, that are usually absent if wax is used instead. The plate being completed, a narrow strip of wax, half an inch wide, must be warmed and bent round to the shape of the dental arch, its thickness varying according to the depth of the bite, that is, the distance between the upper gum and the tops of the lower teeth. On this rim of wax the teeth may be mounted, simply warming them and pressing their fang portion in; when they are all adjusted, (1), with a view to their perfect articulation with their fellows of the lower jaw; (2) with regard to their restoration of the outline of the jaw that has been lost by absorption; and (3) with some display of artistic feeling as to their general appearance and disposition; the spaces surrounding them may be filled in with wax, on the labial surface, being made continuous with the remains of the gums, and on the lingual surface continuous with the palate. On the outer surface avoid a smoothness and continuity that is never found in the natural state, and which, if present, shows a want of taste in the finished piece ; and on the lingual surface avoid depressions and sharp ridges or boundaries that will allow of the lodgment of food, and induce irritation in the tongue. Bear in mind that what the wax is, such will the perfected piece be in these respects, and that as a matter of economy in time and materials what you desire the finished piece to be, that also the wax model should be. Convenient instruments for modelling up the wax around the teeth are shown in the woodcut below (Fig. 78).

FIG. 78.

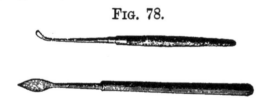

Flasking is the next step. Opinions differ as to the best form of flask to use, but for an upper set of teeth there is little doubt that shown in the annexed cut is the most serviceable (Fig. 79).

FIG. 79.

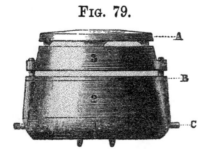

This flask is made after a pattern designed
by Messrs Bell and Turner, in three sections
(Nos 1, 2, 3), and is constructed for the purpose
of avoiding the evils complained of in the old
kinds, viz. that of leaving a stratum of vulcanite between the two halves of the mould, and
thus altering the articulation of the piece ; and
not only this, but causing often a derangement
of the arch or position of the teeth, through
the difficulty of getting the two halves of the
mould to shut down in their proper position.

By the use of the intervening plate B (the
invention of Mr Bennett) an exact fac-simile of
the palate of the patient can be produced upon
the external surface of the vulcanite piece.

If any of the accompanying descriptions of

FIG. 80.

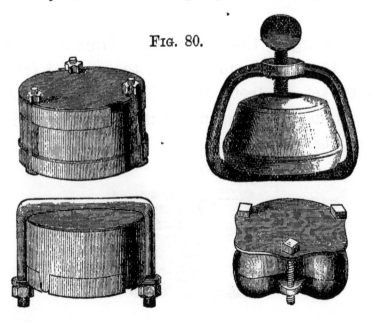

flasks are used (Fig. 80), then the model must be what is called "sunk" in the lower portion thus, (Fig. 81), so that the plaster rises

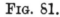

FIG. 81.

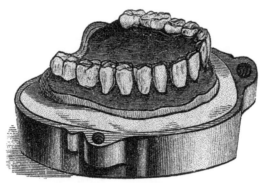

to the level of the wax around the model, not higher. The plaster must be mixed thin, and the model pressed firmly down, in order that it may rest upon the floor of the flask; when it is hard, paint it over with soap and water, by means of a camel's-hair brush, teeth, plaster, and wax altogether, or dust it on the surface, when dry and hard, with soapstone (French chalk) : this is to prevent adhesion of the plaster when the upper part of the flask is filled in. This upper part must now be fitted on, the top being taken off, so that plaster may be poured in from above, and well shaken down, to avoid any air bubbles getting between, what will presently be, the mould and counterpart; when the space is thoroughly filled up, the top piece may be put on, and the whole, while the plaster is soft, put into " the wrench " shown below, so as to ensure all the parts of the flask being in

FIG. 82.

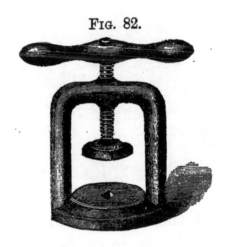

accurate and complete contact, any superfluous plaster being wiped away from the outside of the flask in order to see that this, is accomplished. Or the method of flasking the piece as directed at p. 197 may be adopted which in many cases has advantages over that just described.

Opening the flask must be delayed until the plaster is quite hard; it can then be removed from the wrench, and placed in a basin of boiling water, the joints prised apart with the edge of a knife or scorper, and the separation made between the upper and lower parts; care must be taken to open the flask evenly all round, or there is a liability of breaking away some portion of the plaster.

To clear away the wax.—Pour boiling water over the upper portion of the flask—in which the teeth will be found imbedded—until every particle, and even the appearance of gloss, is gone from the surface of the mould.

Packing may now be proceeded with. The rubber cut up into sizes suitable for the case should be warmed on a hot water-plate (Fig. 83). Packing is not a matter of so much

FIG. 83.

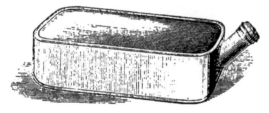

importance as having the rubber thoroughly softened and very clean, so that it may be packed closely together and have no dirt or sulphur on the surface to prevent perfect cohesion of the whole mass. The same description of instrument may be used for packing as for modelling. If more than one sort of rubber is used, care must be taken to keep the line of union as true as possible, so as to prevent a

patchy appearance in the finished case. Packing should always be commenced in that part
which will tend to keep the teeth most firmly
in position. This in most instances will be
close down by the pins of the teeth, as shown
in Fig. 84. When there appears to be sufficient

FIG. 84.

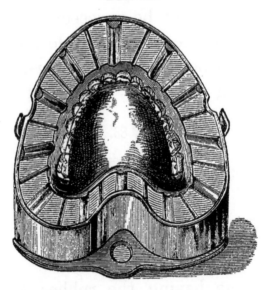

rubber to fill up the mould thoroughly, place it
in the wrench fitted to a celluloid base tank
(Fig. 85), and having boiling water in the tank,
keep up the temperature with the spirit lamp
or gas, and gradually close the flask as far as it
will go without great pressure, then remove it,
immerse for a minute in cold water, and open,
if there is not sufficient rubber put in more, if

there is excess, as there should be, then cut gutters round, as shown in Fig. 84; this will allow the superfluous rubber to flow out when it is again put in the wrench, and enable you to close the flask completely.

FIG. 85.

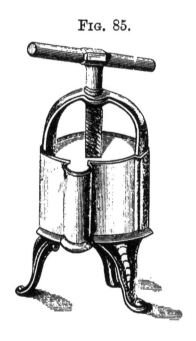

The great advantage in using the celluloid tank is, that it enables you to warm the rubber and flask, and apply the wrench simultaneously.

The benefit derived from the plan of screwing up, before cutting the gutters, is that you press the rubber well home into all the deeper portions of the mould, and also well around the teeth.

To facilitate the opening of the flask for

12

examining the quantity of rubber, a piece of unsized cloth, such as that usually placed between the layers of rubber when sold, only with the size washed out of it, may be interposed between the surface of the rubber and the plaster counter-part. This prevents adhesion of those surfaces, and does not interfere with the perfect union of the pieces of rubber. Care must be taken to remove the cloth before finally screwing up.

Some authors advise coating the plaster with French chalk, liquid silex, collodion, or tinfoil, to prevent adhesion to the rubber; for my own part I prefer leaving the plaster untouched, as anything that is applied will give to the surface of the rubber when hardened, a smooth surface, that is very objectionable if you want to obtain suction; and the plaster adhering to the exposed portion of the plate—that must be finished with file and scraper—is of no consequence.

When the piece is packed and ready for vulcanizing, it must be fitted into its proper clamp, or ring, to secure it, or if it has screws attached, they must be brought home to prevent any chance of gaping, when the rubber begins to swell in the vulcanizer.

Vulcanizers are so numerous that it is somewhat difficult to make a choice; the

most carefully made and perfectly finished
are those manufactured by Messrs Ash; the
least expensive and most ingenious are those
supplied by Messrs White, of Philadelphia;
the simplest is that made by G. W. Rutterford,
of this city, and known as the " *Single-screw
vulcanizer.*" There are many other makers, but
these three indicate the chief characteristics
belonging to their several manufactures. We
will speak of Ash's first (Fig. 86).

FIG. 86.

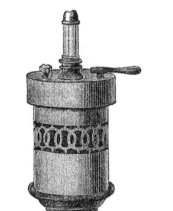

Dimensions : height 15 in., diameter 5¼ in.

The vulcanizing chamber is made of *wrought*
copper, nearly a quarter of an inch thick, and
the *malleable* iron cover is held down by means

of a strong *wrought*-iron screw collar with set screws.

The thermometer registers 350° Fahrenheit, and the small fusible metal plug inserted in the cover will only blow out when that degree of heat is exceeded.

The vulcanizers are tested, before leaving their factory, to a pressure of upwards of 600 lbs. to the square inch, or nearly *seven* times the degree of pressure usually required in the process of vulcanization. An iron ring with handle is with each vulcanizer, to hold the boiler while screwing on the wrought-iron screw collar. It is useful also for turning out the flask when the vulcanizing is complete. The india-rubber packing requires renewing occasionally to keep the chamber steam-tight.

Fig 87.

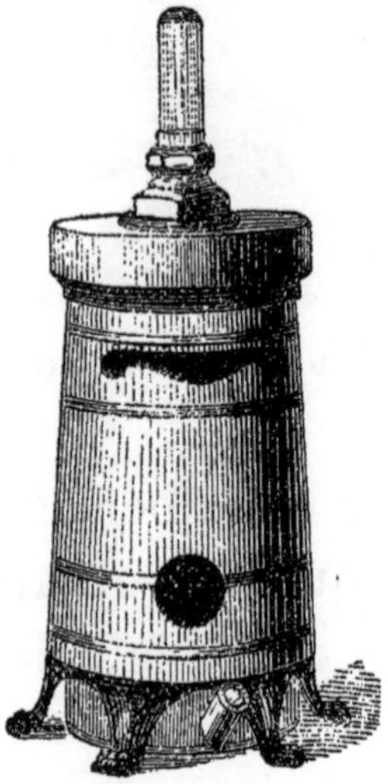

Of the American vulcanizers, Whitney's are, all things considered, the best for ordinary use, and the accompanying woodcut (Fig. 87) shows the most convenient size for general purposes.

The heater is composed entirely of copper and brass, is of two pieces only, a copper pot, and brass head that screws on to the pot, dispensing with all bolts and nuts. They are uniformly $3\frac{7}{8}$ inches diameter inside; for two flasks 5 inches, and for three flasks 7 inches deep. The whole thing complete for use only weighs from 4 to $5\frac{1}{4}$ pounds, according to the size, whether for two or three flasks. Special directions for using accompany each machine.

A small vulcanizer (Fig. 89), known as Hayes'

FIG. 88.

FIG. 89.

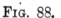
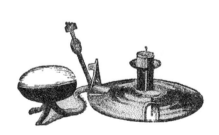
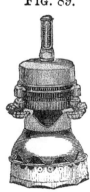

iron-clad, is very useful in travelling or when there is not gas conveniently near; it is made for either one or two flasks, but for real con-

venience the single flask oven is the best;
with this the automatic lamp is very good,
as it will shut off the spirit when the steam is
getting up too high (Fig. 88).

This automatic lamp may be used for gas or

FIG. 90.

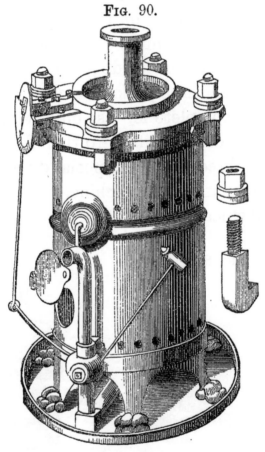

Vulcanizer.

alcohol, and with or without the automatic arrangement.   When properly adjusted the flow of
gas or alcohol is controlled by a spring cut-off,

that is held open by a fusible alloy that breaks loose and extinguishes the flames when the heat reaches a point slightly above that required to finish the process, and before the work or the vessel can receive injury. The wick, being protected from combustion, does not require renewal.

A very complicated, but perfect, apparatus,

FIG. 91.

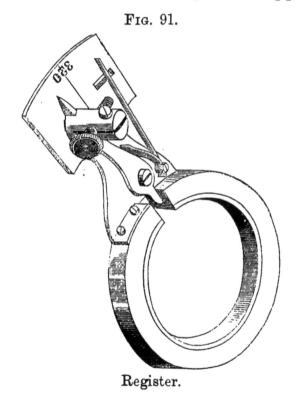

Register.

whereby the thermometer is dispensed with entirely, is shown in the accompanying drawings (Figs. 90, 91), and is known as Hoffstadt's self-regulating vulcanizer.

Many attempts have been made to regulate the flame used for heating vulcanizing machines, and in this vulcanizer the flame is not only regulated as desired, but the degree of heat indicated without a thermometer, and the attention of the operator drawn by the tap of a bell when the heat has reached any given point. The boiler is very strong indeed. A brass ring is well brazed on the outside of the boiler; the lid, which is made of bell-metal, is fastened to the boiler with three hook-shaped screws made of steel. There is a ring cast solid with the outside of the lid, which encloses the inner ring or regulator, that will expand or contract by changes of heat, and work the lever which extends on the platform. The lever comes in contact with the hand on the dial registering the degree of heat, and when the heat has reached any determined point—say 320°—it disconnects the lever which is attached to a spring stop-cock, and turns down the flame as far as the set-screw allows, which may be set to any desired point.

Rutterford's single-screw vulcanizer has a wrought-copper boiler, dome-shaped lid held down by one screw in the centre; the case supporting the boiler is of sheet iron, with cast-iron stand and screw holes to fix it to the work-bench.

The steam is let off at a separate escape-screw, thus leaving the safety-valve undisturbed; there is also a steam-gauge as well as thermometer attached; it can be used, as seen in woodcut (Fig. 92), for either gas or spirit lamp.

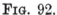

FIG. 92.

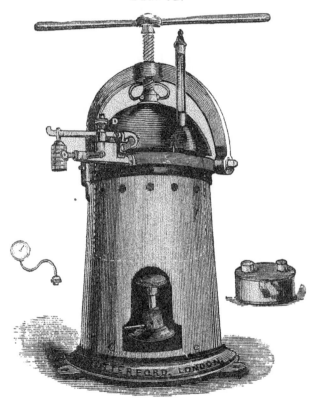

The engraving shows clearly the manner in which it is closed by means of the double ended lever.

The choice of a vulcanizer having been settled, the flask should be placed as near the centre as possible, resting, if there be room, on some pieces of pumice-stone. The amount of water must vary according to the size of the boiler, but with Rutterford's medium-sized vulcanizer I put in half a pint of warm water. When the vulcanizer is closed the heat must be gradually raised—the slower the better—and kept at the temperature required for the necessary time; for most rubbers the best heat is 310° for an hour and a half; if you lengthen the time, you may reduce the heat to 305°; if you raise the heat you may shorten the time proportionately. This latter plan should only be adopted, however, under some great emergency, such as for a hurried repair.

When the time of vulcanization is completed, if possible let the boiler cool down before letting off the steam and opening, as this gradual reduction of temperature tempers the piece better than if you take it out suddenly and cool down with water.

If on opening the vulcanizer, the flask is not quite cold, it may be placed under a tap, and a stream of water allowed to run over it; the screws can then be loosened, or the clamp or ring released, and a thin-edged knife introduced between the joints of the flask, and the parts gradually separated all round, or the top

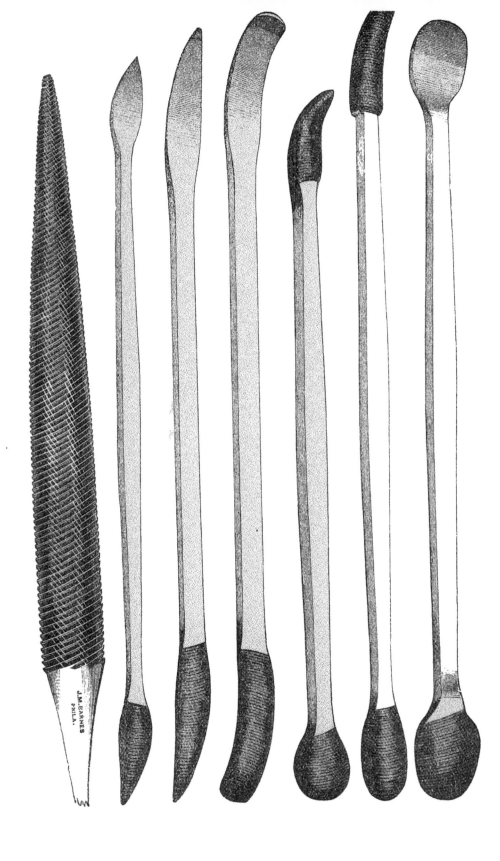

J.M.EARNES
PHILA.

piece may be taken off first of all, and water allowed to soak through so as to soften the plaster. In opening either way, however, the only thing required is care and attention, with the recollection of the position the teeth occupy in the flask. After taking out the piece, cleanse it thoroughly with cold water and a good stiff tooth or nail brush so as to free it from plaster. As it is now ready for filing up, with straight and curved rough files remove the superfluous rubber, and reduce all the surface (except the interior, which is to fit the gums and palate) to their proper thickness and size and shape. The files best suited for this purpose are shown in Fig. 93.

A quicker, but somewhat dangerous plan, is to thin down the piece with a burr or steel wheel (file-cut) on the lathe. There is, however, an obvious risk of cutting through the palatine portion of the plate unless great care is used. The cut, Fig. 94, shows the burrs made by Messrs Ash to fit on the lathe heads manufactured by them.

An even surface having been obtained by one or other of these means, the vulcanite must be cleared away from around the teeth, so as to give the outline of the artificial gum as natural an appearance as possible. This is best done

FIG. 94.

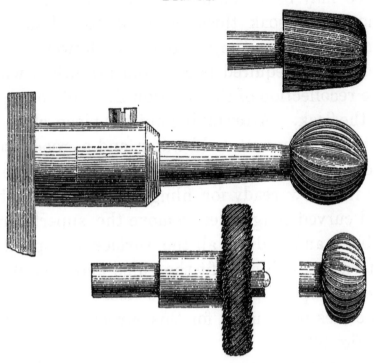

by means of scorpers, or sculptors as they are also called, the drawing shows them in plane and in section, the various forms being used according to the position of the rubber to be removed by them.

The plate having been filed up is ready for "finishing," that is, reduced to a smooth surface by means of scrapers, fine files, glass cloth, pumice powder, and lathe. Some very useful forms of scrapers are shown in woodcut, Fig. 95. They are capable, however, of very many modifications, according to the skill and fancy

FIG. 95.

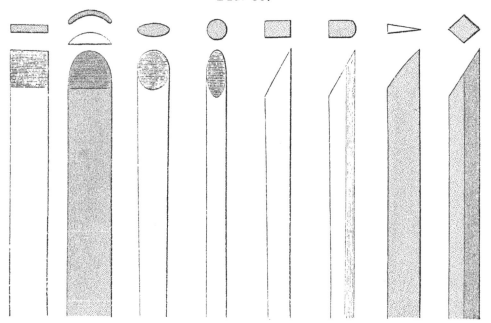

of the operator. These various shapes it will be seen are made with a view to fit into the different parts of an artificial denture. Many will finish up with the scraper and glass cloth alone, and then lathe with pumice, while others prefer to use Ayrstone, after the glass clothing, using a fine file also with the scraper to improve the surface. Some, again, like to go over the entire surface with a stick, and water and pumice powder, to take out all the scratches. All these different plans are matters of individual taste. The only thing to be remembered is this, that you must have all the scratches

FIG. 96.

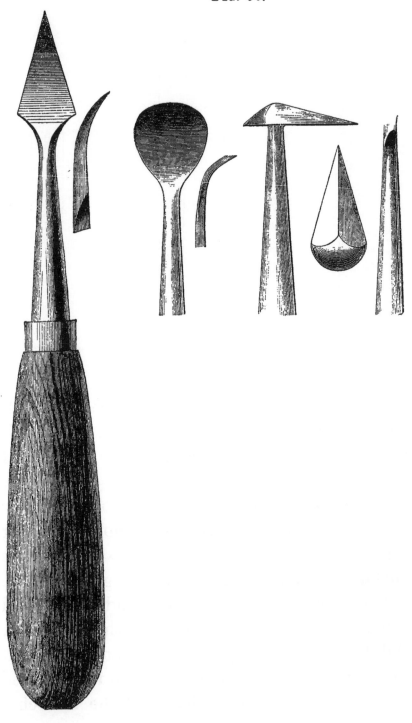

out by one means or other before you begin
polishing at the lathe wheel. The best arranged
polishing lathe is shown in Fig. 97. The

FIG. 97.

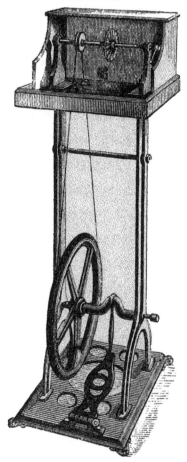

splashings are prevented from scattering about,
and there is plenty of room for the hands to
move the plate of rubber in all directions.
When using the pumice powder and hard brush
for polishing be careful to have plenty of water;

13

this gives a better finish in shorter time. When a smooth continuous surface has been obtained, change the hard brush for a soft one, or an American buff wheel or cone, and proceed with whiting and water to put on the finishing polish.   To do this use plenty of water at first, and then complete the process by working the brush till it is dry; by these means I have always obtained the best results.   Some use after this, crocus and oil as a final surface polish.   I prefer, however, using only the whiting.   Last of all, cleanse the piece carefully with warm water and soap, using a soft brush, and it is ready for fitting in the mouth.

A full lower set can of course be made in precisely similar fashion to an upper set.   I shall, therefore, now go on to treat of—

Partial cases (for the upper jaw).   The upper and lower models with their articulations, we shall take for granted are complete.   The teeth must then be in most cases fitted to the gum very carefully, so that there may be no rubber likely to show underneath, when the piece is finished.   If the bite is very close it may be necessary to use plate teeth; then unless the pins are very long and strong, it will be wiser to strengthen them by means of a strip of gold soldered to them, varying the shape of the gold

according to circumstances. For most cases the
forms shown in Figs. 98 and 99 will answer best.
This gives plenty of room for rubber all round,
and holds very firmly. Another way is to
form a loop thus, Fig. 100, or as in Fig. 101, the

FIG. 98.　　　FIG. 99.　　　FIG. 100.　　　FIG. 101.

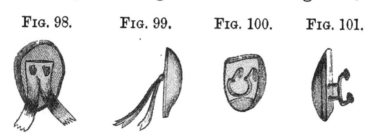

ends being clubbed. It will be seen at once
how much they may be varied to suit the peculiarities of the case. The teeth being fitted
into their places on the model, they may be
attached to the temporary plate made up according to the instructions already given, but
altered in size according to the number of teeth
it is to carry, and whether it is to be kept up
by suction or by bands. If it is necessary to
use bands round some of the teeth to support
the case, gold clasps are the neatest, but I
consider vulcanite the least injurious.

In every artificial denture there is invariably
a certain amount of friction produced by the
movement of the plate in mastication, if gold
is used, the metal, being harder than the tooth,
wears it away; if, on the other hand, vulcanite

is used, that substance, being softer than the tooth, is itself worn away instead; and for these reasons I should advise the use of vulcanite bands, if possible, instead of gold clasps.

If vulcanite bands are necessary they will of course be formed of wax on the model previous to flasking; if clasps of gold are thought desirable they had better be adjusted after fitting the teeth, and may be formed thus :—A strip (varying in width according to the length of the tooth) of clasp gold, about No. 7 gauge,

FIG. 102.

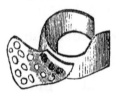

A strip of plate perforated and soldered on.

FIG. 103.

For a canine tooth, three strips soldered together at one point, and then diverged.

FIG. 104.

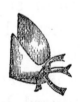

Clubbed strips soldered on and bent up at ends.

FIG. 105.

Club-headed pieces soldered on.

FIG. 106.

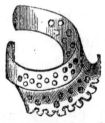

Band drilled and countersunk, the lower edge roughened and bent outwards.

must be bent up to fit the tooth well, after the manner described in the section on gold work; it must then be fitted up so as to have a firm hold in the vulcanite. The annexed cuts show various ways of doing this, according to the space and thickness of rubber you have to surround the clasp.

The teeth and bands having been properly adjusted to the model, and to each other, the case is ready for flasking; one other thing remains to be done, however, that is, to cut down to half their length, the plaster teeth on the model; the object of this will be seen presently. The model and case are now sunk in the lower portion of the flask (into which plaster mixed to the consistence of cream has already been poured). Instead of leaving the teeth exposed, the plaster is carried over so that only the inner surface of the teeth show (Fig. 107). This plan may also be adopted for a full set of teeth, as seen in the drawing given.

By this method displacement of the teeth is almost impossible, at the same time that any accession of rubber in the wrong place (that is, under the teeth) is also prevented. The rest of the process is the same as that already described for a full upper set. Only one caution must be given, and that is, to well bevel the sides

FIG. 107.

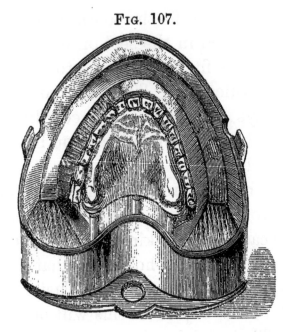

of the overlap of the teeth, so that the central portion, especially the plug, may draw away easily and without the risk of breaking. Partial cases must be made of varying thickness according to the nature of the piece, and may sometimes be strengthened with strips of gold wire flattened, running across any narrow or weak part.

The strengthening of a vulcanite plate may be advisable sometimes in either the upper or under jaw. For the upper it generally occurs when, from the thinness you desire to have the plate or the conformation of the arch, there occurs greater liability to fracture than usual, from the increased strain on weak points.

A strengthener must be made by bending up a strip of gold, one sixteenth of an inch wide, to fit fairly well to the palate from side to side, about opposite the second molars. This must be pierced with holes along its borders. Now take this strip and place it edgeways upon another piece of plate, and trace the outline of its concave surface. Draw another line one sixteenth of an inch beyond this again, and cut up the pattern indicated by the lines; you will then have two pieces of the annexed form (Fig. 108). It is evident now that the convex *edge* of A will

Fig. 108.

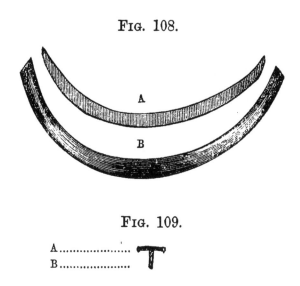

Fig. 109.

A....................
B....................

fit on to the concave *surface* of B, and being placed in the centre of B the two may be soldered together. Now, if we look at them in section we have this view (Fig. 109), combining at once the greatest strength with the greatest lightness and but small expenditure of material, while at the same time we have only the thin edge of A presented on the palate, supposing the workman should be so unfortunate as to file away the rubber to such an extent as to expose it. The size of the two plates of gold can of course vary according to circumstances, but the principle is the same. An identical plan can be adopted for the lower jaw (letting the one plate rest against the natural front teeth, if they are present). By this method we can give to a vulcanite case very great strength and stiffness, without making it much heavier for the mouth. When spiral springs are to be fitted to the set you may even cut all the central portion of the palate away, simply leaving a band of rubber running across the back of the mouth, and strengthened in this way. Lower pieces also may be much reduced in bulk. If this plan is adopted it will at once be seen how much stronger it is than a piece of round wire flattened, or even an ordinary gold plate strengthener. It is also applicable as a means of increasing the strength of teeth, running out alone, on a narrow strip of rubber between large natural teeth.

Repairing vulcanite plates is not very satisfactory, as the second vulcanizing necessarily renders the piece brittle and darker in colour than it naturally should be. The plan adopted in all cases is essentially the same, so that general instructions will be sufficient. In the event of either a fracture of the plate or a tooth being broken off, cut out with a fine saw all the impaired portion of rubber, having of course first secured a model of the mouth. Then cut dovetails into the rubber where union is desired. If it be a lower piece and there is plenty of substance, drill into the surface of the dovetails to give the rubber firmer hold. Now, instead of filling in the gap around the tooth or fracture with wax, use modelling clay, and you will have an equally smooth surface, and when it is vulcanized you will find the joining is scarcely perceptible—a thing that is above all others to be desired by those who take a proper interest in the appearance of their work when finished. When sinking a repair in the flask cover everything but the portion that will require packing, and instead of flasking in the lower portion, use the upper section, first because it is deeper and prevents the risk of the rubber being near the iron and so becoming blackened; and, secondly, because the top taking off it allows of easier removal of the plate after vulcanization is completed.

If there be any discoloration after repairing a piece, it may be removed to some extent, according to Dr Richardson ('Mechanical Dentistry,' p. 42), by " moistening the surface with dilute nitric acid for a short time, after which the piece is thoroughly washed and then placed for a few minutes in an alkaline solution, to remove any remaining traces of acid," or " expose the piece to the rays of the sun in alcohol for five or six hours."

To reset a vulcanite piece.—Make a false model first, by soaping the rubber on the palatine side, pouring in plaster and building up as for an ordinary model ; then round the outside of the plaster cast cut out four grooves horizontally or make two depressions in front of a conical form with a sculpter or knife ; soap or oil all this surface, and the fronts of the teeth as well, and pour over plaster tolerably stiff in substance, so as not to run about easily ; bring this out beyond the model, half an inch in thickness, and let it extend upwards to a level with the cutting edge of the teeth ; we then obtain results shown in Fig. 110. These two portions having been carefully separated may be again put into place, the palate of the piece soaped, as well

Fig. 110.

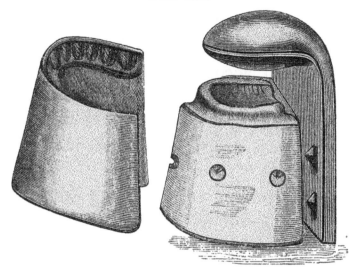

as the top edge of the outer casting, and plaster poured over like a hooded bite.

When these are divided and the piece to be reset taken off the model, it will be seen that we have all the dimensions of the old plate in such a form as to be able to reproduce them with the same teeth but fresh rubber, or if it is for a duplicate case, with another set of teeth, fitting into the same moulds.

Supposing, however, that the piece is simply to be reset, by this plan we avoid the risk of breaking the teeth by taking them out of the old setting of rubber when sunk in the flask, and if an accident should by any chance occur, it is more easily remedied. The castings being completed, the teeth taken off the old plate and cleaned carefully, and the pins readjusted, they are placed in their moulds in the outer casting, connected together with wax, and the rest of the plate filled in according to the space in the moulds; by this mode of procedure any alteration may be made in a piece whilst at the same time we retain exact models of the original form.

From the various ways in which vulcanite can be used it will at once suggest itself as a convenient material to reset ill-fitting gold plates, when from a large amount of absorption of the alveoli the denture can no longer be worn with comfort. Several plans may be adopted in order to ascertain the amount of fresh material that it is required to add to the plate. For either method first perforate the plate, to be refitted, with a number of small holes (tooth pin size is best), choosing for their situation, as far as possible, the borders of the plate; but in addition any spot that indicates a capability of giving good retaining power to the rubber when vulcanized; the most simple and at the same time certain thing to do after this is to fill the hollow portion of the gold plate with plaster of Paris rather thicker than for an ordinary impression, then introduce it into the mouth and tell the patient to close the jaws, and see that the articulation is correct. When the plaster is quite hard remove it, soap the surface and cast in the lower part of a flask, as if it were an ordinary impression, then trim off the burrs of plaster that have worked through the perforations, coat over any irregularities with wax, if necessary, soap the whole and fill in the upper part of the flask as for an ordinary case; when hard separate carefully; the gold plate and teeth will now be found in all probability in the upper part of the flask, separated from the plaster impression; this latter must be prised off, the holes in the plate cleaned of wax or plaster with boiling water, and packing may then be proceeded with in the usual manner. If there are tube teeth on the case they must be taken off previously to the sinking of the plate, and fixed on again afterwards with floss silk and mastic; if only backed teeth are on the case it need give no extra trouble of this sort.

Another plan consists of taking a model and articulation, then lining the plate with wax or gutta percha and pressing on the *model* instead of in the mouth to obtain indications of the parts to be refitted; it will at once be seen, however, that the first-mentioned method is infinitely better if carefully carried out.

The impression having been obtained in the

plastic material, the remaining portion of the process is of course identical with the one first described.

A third plan is to place the plate upon the model and seal the edges where they are not close to the model, to prevent the ingress of plaster. The model with the piece upon it is now sunk in the flask, keeping the gold case quite clear of plaster, so that it will readily leave the model and be included in the other half of the flask. Into the non-fitting parts of the plate rubber is placed and vulcanized, having previously prepared the plate to hold it, either by soldering small pieces thereto, or by roughening the plate with a pointed instrument. By this mode there is no trouble required in modelling up the plate with wax, &c. ; but where the whole surface of a plate has to be covered with vulcanite, and the articulation of the piece consequently altered, either of the methods previously described will be found more applicable.

When the rubber is vulcanized to gold and it is necessary to bevel off the plate at any part to make it continuous with the rubber, do not file the plate, but grind at the lathe with a very fine wheel. In this way you will avoid the danger of turning up the thin edge of gold that your grinding has produced. With the file great trouble sometimes occurs in getting a smooth surface where the gold and rubber join.

For lower and partial cases the same rules will of course apply as for an upper set.

To improve the colour of vulcanized rubber it may be placed in a glass covered vessel containing alcohol, and set in the sun for six or eight hours ; the longer the time (in reason) the better the colour will be.

SECTION XI

THE CELLULOID BASE

THE Albany Dental Plate Company in 1871 took out patents and sent over specimens of a new base for artificial teeth. The composition is said to consist of solid collodion, prepared in a peculiar manner. It is really gun-cotton and camphor, and from the specification we learn that " in the manufacture of collodion for these dental plates the inventors prefer to use at least fifty parts by weight of gum camphor to one hundred parts of soluble cotton (a greater proportion of camphor may be used), whereby the product is rendered more plastic than when a less quantity is employed. The collodion thus produced is made into plates of suitable thickness, which are preferably formed into shapes approximating to those of finished dental plates by pressure in heated moulds. The plates thus formed are now thoroughly dried by placing them in a drying-room heated to a temperature which should not exceed 180° Fah.,

150° to 180° being the temperature found best adapted for expelling the camphor solvent. A temperature much higher than 200° will expand the material, and render it porous and brittle. The plates when properly dried, although freed from liability of shrinkage, still retain the quality which enables them to become plastic under a proper degree of heat, and may be readily moulded into any desired shape without subsequently shrinking to any injurious extent."

There are two varieties,—the coloured, which is of a gum-like pink; and the uncoloured, which is semi-transparent, and of an amber-yellow.

We will first take the properties of the two, and then their application to dental purposes.

Both are in their uncorked state stronger and lighter than any dental rubber. The uncoloured celluloid is, however, stronger and lighter than the pink, but the amber-coloured base is more liable to warp than the pink.

In opposition to the statement contained in the circular sent out, I must say that in my experience both kinds are affected by the acids of the mouth : the uncoloured, instead of remaining semi-transparent, assumes an opaque appearance, becomes much harder, and is dis-

14

coloured by blood; while the pink, after a few weeks' wear, has a white granulated look over the surface. These changes, however, do not affect the durability of the piece.

It has a strong smell, and a slight taste of camphor, which remains for five or six days; it is not, however, as a rule, objected to by patients, and to many is not even unpleasant.

To remove the smell of the camphor, if it should be found objectionable, the piece may be placed for four or five hours in a solution consisting of sulphuric acid one part, and water two parts, a larger proportion of acid affecting the piece injuriously. This suggestion I give on the authority of the inventors.

With *Chlorætherine* it is converted into a soft gelatinous mass, but is not dissolved; and as the chlorætherine evaporates, it again becomes hard. With *Sulphuric ether* the surfaces of two pieces may be softened, and, being kept in contact for three or four hours, will become as one. Pieces cannot be softened so as to unite together by dry heat.

The older the plates are when received from the depôts the stronger they appear, and the less liable to shrink; this, I think, is owing to the evaporation of a portion of the camphor which they contain. All parts brought into contact with metal of any kind become white and opaque more quickly than the rest of the piece.

Pieces may be softened and allowed to harden any reasonable number of times without apparent deterioration of texture. The temperature of the mouth does not affect it injuriously, but the heat of boiling water will soften it. Boiled for ten hours in water it becomes deprived of a large portion of its camphor, and remains a white friable mass.

As to the mode of using it, I do not think we have arrived at anything like perfection, nor even do we yet know the simplest way of applying it.

The plan I at present adopt is, after sinking the pieces made up on wax in the flask, as if for vulcanite, to choose the base of an approximate size, cutting away any portions that may appear in excess, and then softening the celluloid sufficiently in boiling fluid to enable it to be pressed into shape in the flask with the fingers; the two parts of the flask can be brought more closely together at the beginning, and there is less risk of injuring the plaster castings. When the flask is nearly closed I open it, and cut out gutters for the excess that may be present. This plan insures plenty of the base being pressed well round the teeth, and into any overlaps that the piece may have.

Gutters having been freely cut, the flask may be completely closed, after the heat has been increased sufficiently, and then the whole taken out of the tank and placed in cold water, where it should remain for twenty minutes, or it may remain in the tank for ten minutes, thus cooking it more completely.

The best flask, clamp, and tank for the purpose are those recommended and sold at the depôts, as being made by White, of Philadelphia (Fig. 111); the principal feature and advantage

FIG. 111.

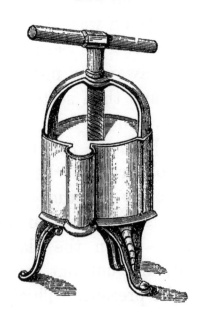

being that the flask can be gradually closed while it is in the boiling fluid, which cannot be done in the ordinary way.

As to the fluid in which the piece should be softened, I think oil the best; it is not so injurious to the celluloid as I consider water to be, and it toughens the plates. Dry heat I believe to be unsatisfactory. The plaster for the flasks, if mixed tolerably stiff, is quite strong enough without the addition of any substance, such as gum-arabic; in fact, in using water alone the plaster becomes so hard as to be difficult of removal from the flask. To prevent the base adhering, the castings may be painted over with oil, or dusted over with French chalk. The piece can be finished up in the ordinary way with scraper, file, and glass-paper, or, better than glass-paper, at the lathe with a wet hard brush, plenty of water, and coarse pumice, afterwards whiting and oil, and finally a dry felt cone with dry whiting, or, according to White's circular, the dry cone alone. It may be repaired in the same way as vulcanite, by dovetailing; but I do not think the pieces, as a rule, become thoroughly welded; this, I believe, can only be perfectly done by means of a solvent. By immersion in boiling fluid any part of it can be altered in form, in the same manner as vulcanite, and should afterwards be put into cold water to thoroughly re-harden.

At present I have no great faith in its use for repairing vulcanite—there is simply mechanical union ; and, as the two substances are of such very different density, they do not hold very firmly even when thoroughly dovetailed.

After a series of experiments, carefully conducted, with the celluloid base, I have obtained the following results :—

Taking first the essential oils :—Two grains of the base reduced by filing to a fine state of division, were placed in a test-tube containing *Oil of Cassia*, and the result was a transparent gelatinous mass, insoluble with heat. With *Oil of Cloves* we found the same action ; with *Oil of Rosemary* a slightly gelatinous condition was seen to be present, but it was not soluble ; and with *Oil of Origanum* it was not acted upon at all.

In *Benzole, rectified spirits of wine, pure Ether,* and *Potassium Naphtha*, it was quite insoluble. It is but very slightly soluble in *Chlorform*, and it is not acted upon at all by *Thymol* in any of its forms.

By the action of *Creosote*, when heated, it shows a mass in a gelatinous form suspended in the liquid; and in *Carbolic acid* we have the same conditions, only more strongly marked.

If placed in a vessel containing any of the fatty oils, and heated up to their boiling-point, it is completely decomposed, leaving only a residue of carbon; the same thing happens if heated alone in a test-tube, the camphor being driven off, and leaving carbon behind. In fact, the application of great heat (especially dry heat) causes the camphor to be driven off, and tends to the rapid disintegration of the compound.

I have brought forward the results of these experiments, because I think that the celluloid base may be prepared in such a way as to be most useful for a temporary stopping; it is therefore important that we should have some knowledge of the action of those preparations with which it might be brought into contact in a tooth, as, for instance, *Carbolic acid, Thymol,* and others.

From the comparative facility with which the celluloid can be prepared, and the ease with which it can be produced in any colour, I have fair hope we may obtain some temporary stoppings of great value for many cases. This, however, is a matter for future consideration.

I consider the base a useful introduction, but not one of great value at present; still, it is so good that I believe it is capable and worthy of improvement.

For artificial dentures it is comfortable and light to wear, the pink is natural in appearance, and it adapts itself well to the mouth; how it will last, time alone can show. At present it is most available for pieces intended only for temporary wear, from the fact, as an American writer amusingly puts it, that the teeth have a tendency to shed.

SECTION XII

THE TREATMENT OF DEFORMITIES OF THE MOUTH

THE Dental Surgeon is occasionally called upon to treat certain deformities of the mouth quite distinct from those malformations that may arise from irregularity of the teeth. These I have fully entered into in my work on that subject published by the Messrs Churchill. In the following section I shall therefore condense what I have already written upon the subject in the volume referred to.

Deformities of the mouth arise from three distinct causes,—congenital deficiency, as in cleft palate ; perforation and lesion of the hard or soft palate, and sometimes both, from phagædenic or syphilitic ulceration ; or in the third place from mechanical injury, such as gunshot wounds, or injury arising from any other form of violence.

We will consider first the treatment of CONGENITAL CLEFT PALATE.

Taking the Impression.—The materials generally used for taking impressions of the mouth are by no means satisfactory, in taking impressions of parts that are so easily displaced as the soft palate, for none of them can be used, under the most favorable circumstances, without applying pressure sufficient to render the impression and model incorrect.

It being, then, necessary to introduce some preparation into the mouth in such a state that it will not move the most delicate fold of mucous membrane, while in a short time it shall become so hard as to admit of removal without any alteration of form, I recommend plaster of Paris.

In most cases the soft palate will be found too sensitive at first to admit of a full impression being taken at once, or even of the holding of the impression plate in position sufficiently long to admit of a model being taken. Two courses are open to the operator to overcome this difficulty: one is to take an impression first of only the front of the mouth and cleft and then on successive occasions gradually extend it backwards, till at last you are enabled to get a good impression of the whole of the parts, extending outwards to the alveolar ridge, upwards to the remains of the vomer, and backwards to the posterior wall of the pharynx and pillars of the fauces. Another method is to paint the parts with a solution of bromide of ammonia or tannin and glycerine, ʒi to ʒiv applied with a camel's-hair brush—of the form shown in Fig. 112,* the brush acting almost as beneficially as the preparation used.

FIG. 112.

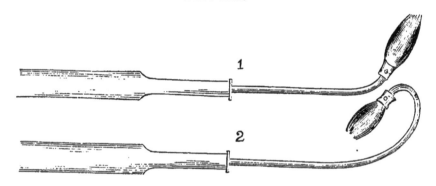

One or other of these two plans must be adopted before any hope can be entertained of getting a good impression. When the parts are rendered sufficiently insensible to the presence of a foreign body, an impression-tray must be carefully prepared, so as to fit in front closely to the teeth, and at the back part leave a space about the eighth of an inch in extent from its surface to the corresponding surface of the soft palate. This does away with the necessity of an excess of plaster, and the consequent risk of any portion falling into the

* Made by Meyer and Metzler, of Great Portland Street.

throat or upon the base of the tongue, and thus produce such irritation that the utmost self-control on the part of the patient will scarcely be able to overcome it.

I have found that a good plan is to use a tray of the form of a common spoon, that I have had made for me by the Messrs Ash and Sons, of Broad Street. These being of pewter, can be bent about to the desired form and then covering with sheet gutta percha, which is placed on the tray and put into the mouth while warm. In this manner you get the outline of the teeth, which will act as a guide in introducing the tray with the plaster on it.

For an ordinary impression of cleft palate, where there is plenty of room to pass the plaster in and out of the mouth, the plate being prepared for use, the next step is the mixing of the plaster; and here several considerations must be taken into account—(1) the dryness of the plaster, (2) its strength, and (3) the time it takes to set, which will depend partly on its freshness, and partly on the temperature of the atmosphere, as well as the water with which it is mixed.

The best plan is to have the water with just the chill off, and then add salt in the proportion of as much as will lie upon a sixpence to half a pint of water. If you wish the plaster to set quicker than under these circumstances it would do, add to it before mixing a small portion of rouge. This will make it set so quickly, and so strongly, that increased care and watchfulness will be required with regard to the proper time for removal from the mouth. Everything being ready, the plaster is mixed in the ordinary manner to the consistence of thick cream, care of course being taken to break up all lumps in it during mixing; a sufficient quantity is then placed in or upon the impression-plate, and the whole steadily introduced into the mouth and held firmly in its place, the precaution being adopted at the moment of putting the plate in position to incline the patient's head forward, so as not only to get a good overlap above the anterior margin of the cleft, but also to lessen the liability of any plaster running down backwards and causing retching.

When the remains of the unused plaster in the bowl will break asunder and leave a clean, sharp fracture, then it is time to remove the impression from the mouth. If at the first it cannot be disengaged easily, then at once and without any hesitation use sufficient force to detach it, bearing in mind that at such a time every second's delay increases the difficulty.

Under ordinary circumstances it will break away in the line of the cleft. This need occasion no alarm : only desire your patient to sit perfectly still and keep the mouth well open ; you can then without any anxiety or hurry push the part which remains above the margin of the palate carefully backwards to the widest part of the opening, and, firmly seizing it with a pair of long tweezers (as shown in Fig 113), withdraw it.

FIG. 113.

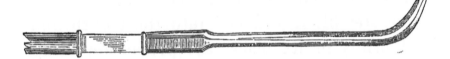

The entire length of these tweezers is eleven inches with the handle.*

The fractured parts, when put carefully together, will be found quite as efficient for use as if no breakage had taken place, especially if, instead of using resin and wax cement, they are united with liquid silex, as recommended in the 'British Journal of Dental Science' for June, 1868,† by which means any increase of bulk is avoided.

* Made by Messrs Ash and Sons, Broad Street, Golden Square.
† "Liquid Silex." By Oakley Coles.

The impression, being thus perfect, must be carefully washed over with a solution of soap (brown Windsor is the best for the purpose), and the model made in three portions, as shown in the accompanying engraving (Fig. 114). We

FIG. 114.

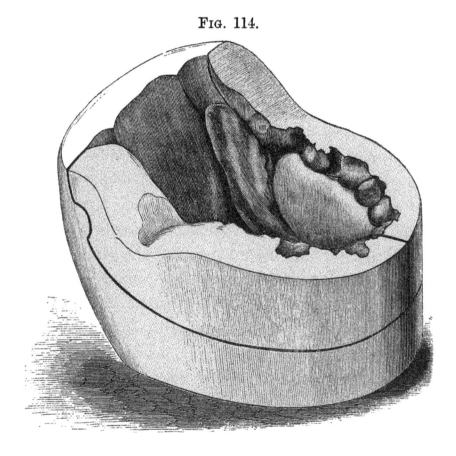

now return to the more commonplace operations of the work-room, and further minute particulars would only become tedious and unnecessary. See section on Modelling.

The model being ready for use, the artificial velum must be set up in gutta percha, having the precise shape which it will possess in its finished form. Here instruction is useless, as the formation of the palate-piece will depend entirely on the characteristics of the case and the ingenuity of the operator. The gutta percha should be of the best description, and the model prepared with soapstone, to prevent any adhesion to its surface. When this is worked up to a satisfactory state, the casting of the plaster moulds can be proceeded with. For an ordinary case the best form is that shown in the engraving (Fig. 115). These, however, admit of very many modifications, according to the shape of the velum, in preparation. The plaster castings, when complete, must be duplicated in type metal, the best metal obtainable and the finest casting-sand only being used. Great care must be taken here, as an imperfection in the metallic moulds will be communicated to the surface of the rubber during vulcanizing, and can only be remedied by clipping and paring, which gives a very unsightly appearance to the finished work. When the castings are complete, and the surfaces well polished with pumice powder and water by means of a stick of dog-wood, they should fit

FIG. 115.

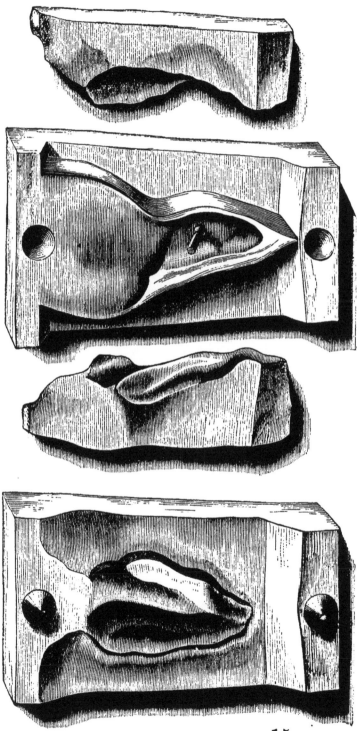

together accurately ; if they do not, there is no alternative but to commence *de novo* till you arrive at a satisfactory result.

The accompanying engraving (Fig. 115) shows the castings separated, also the metallic pin fixed in the base for producing the hole in the velum by which it is attached to the hard rubber front piece. Any error with this will be found to upset the entire arrangement. The greatest care must therefore be used in getting it into a good position, according to the shape of the cleft and mouth. The moulds having been well soaped to prevent adhesion, and made warm— not hot—the next step is to pack them with elastic rubber. This is very easily accomplished : the two side-pieces, being adjusted to the base, are kept firmly in position by an iron clamp, and the rubber packed in from above. When there appears sufficient, the top is put on, and the whole screwed tightly together, being put on a hot plate for a few minutes to soften the rubber. The casts are then taken apart, any excess removed, or any deficiency filled up. They are again screwed up and fitted in an iron framework, as shown in Fig. 116, with wedges to secure them, and put into the vulcanizer. In reference to the rubber to be used, there can be no question that which is

FIG. 116.

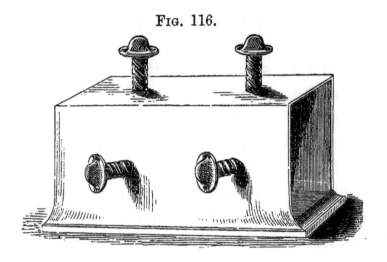

prepared by Messrs Ash and Sons is by far the best, both as regards quality of materials and wear.

The time for vulcanizing this description of rubber is six hours ; that is to say—

2 hours at 240°.
2 hours at 250°.
2 hours at 260°.

An artificial velum will then be produced of the greatest elasticity and power of resistance to the acids of the mouth. It has occasionally been a subject of inquiry as to the description of vulcanizer I use ; I may therefore state that I prefer Rutterford's Single-screw vulcanizer.

The adjustment of a front piece to keep the velum in the cleft will depend on the state of the teeth. If they are all perfect, a simple suction-plate is all that is necessary. If any teeth should be wanting, artificial ones to supply their place should be mounted on the front piece, as in an ordinary set of teeth ; and if there be any deformity of the hard palate, as in most cases there is when associated with harelip, it will have to be restored and made as symmetrical as possible by additions to the hard rubber. When, however, the anterior portion of the mouth is perfect, the palate should be made as thin as possible, and not extend further back than the second bicuspids.

The pin for connecting it with the elastic velum should be of soft platina wire, larger at the top so as to prevent it coming out of the hole in the artificial palate easily; that portion which goes into the hard rubber front piece may be either notched and roughened by the file or have a small piece of plate soldered to it at a right angle, so as to hold it firmly in place.

The following cases will give examples of the various forms of instruments that may be used to remedy a cleft palate according to its peculiar conformation.

The object has been in every instance to close, by means of an artificial palate, the defect in the mouth, and at the same time to

offer every possible chance to a natural effort
to reduce the size of the opening, and not
under any circumstances to enlarge the cleft.

John T—, æt. 4.—Brought to me July,
1868, with fissure of the soft palate and partly
of the hard palate also.   After some little
trouble an impression was obtained, and an
artificial palate fitted in as shown in the
accompanying woodcut, Fig. 117.

FIG. 117.

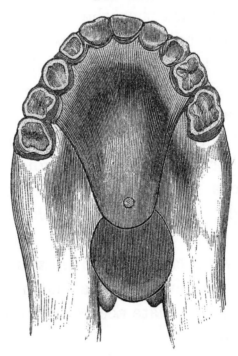

The object and result of fitting in an artificial
palate at this early age is to reduce the size of

the cleft, and so ultimately render the voice less indistinct than it would be if allowed to go on untreated.

When the cleft is left open, every act of swallowing, by the pressure exerted against the margins of the divided palate, tends to more widely separate them; but if an elastic flap covers the opening, the pressure tends to flatten out the bundles of muscular fibres on each side and push them towards each other. The instrument in the present case has been in use for nearly two years, and the results are most satisfactory. If it be urged that surgical treatment is ultimately a more satisfactory proceeding, this preparation only gives the surgeon a greater chance of success, and for this reason alone would be wise and justifiable to adopt.

E. A—, æt. 9—, was brought to me October, 1868, with cleft of soft and portion of hard palate; the speech was very bad, and the child had a vacant unintelligent stare; with slight deafness in both ears.

The margins of the cleft were thick and widely separated; under no circumstances did they touch the posterior wall of the pharynx. I deemed this a most favorable opportunity for trying the utmost that could be done in the way of approximating the free borders of the cleft, and also spreading out the muscular fibres towards the posterior part of the pharynx. The front part of the arch of the palate was very deep, the teeth good and perfect.

October 28th I fitted in a hard rubber palate plate, just reaching to the apex of the fissure. Strange to say, and greatly to my astonishment, the voice was immediately improved. This was worn for six or seven months; then I extended the posterior border of the plate over about one fourth of the cleft, but without putting any overlap. The child had got such power of suction in the front portion of it that this was readily kept in place ; every two or three months I increased this flap a little, until at the present time the cleft is / completely closed by the artificial palate. The front piece fits quite easily, and is the original plate made nearly two years ago, simply having the elastic rubber added to it from time to time. There is no overlap to any portion of the cleft, and the plate depends absolutely on suction for its support, not even fitting tightly to the necks of the teeth. When the velum is taken out it is most interesting to watch the movements of the sides of the cleft, the muscular fibres of which are flattened and spread out by the pressure from below of the elastic rubber. They can be approximated so as to come into actual contact, and the apices of the bifid uvula rest against the back of the pharynx as in a mouth without any deformity.

FIG. 118.   FIG. 119.   FIG. 120.

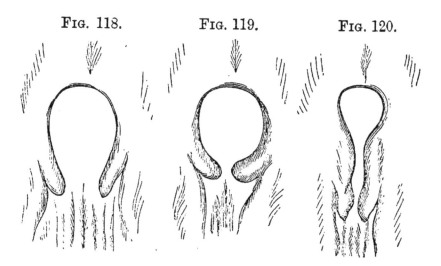

Fig. 118.—Shows the size of the cleft when at rest.

Fig. 119.—Shows the relative position of the parts when they are thrown forward.

Fig. 120.—Shows the "bulging out" and approximation of them towards each other. It. is hardly necessary to add, that the speech has considerably improved during the last year and three quarters, so that the child can go to school and mingle with other children without any difficulty.

W. S—, æt. 17.—Brought to me March, 1869, with cleft of both hard and soft palate, complicated with fissure of the alveolus on the left side.

The appearance of the mouth, when fitted with an artificial velum, and the central and lateral incisor teeth, that had not been developed, is shown in Fig. 121.

FIG. 121.

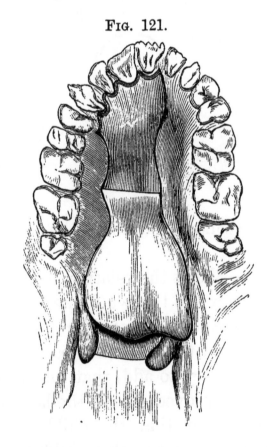

By a mistake in drawing this upon the wood the cleft in the alveolus shows on the right side, whereas it was really on the left, as most of these are.

It will be seen that I have altered the manner in which the hard and soft rubber portions are united together, by giving a continuous flush surface to them, instead of allowing the hard rubber to present a prominent ridge in the centre of the palate. Up to the present time this case has gone on exceedingly satisfactorily.

Miss F—, æt. 17.—Seen by me June, 1868, fair complexion, nervous temperament. There was not much sensitiveness as regards the deformity, and unfortunately no ear for musical sounds, though the young lady played several instruments with ordinary accuracy and ability. There was also slight deafness, probably arising from inflammation of the mucous membrane around the Eustachian tubes, the inflammation having arisen from the great exposure of the parts to every change of temperature in consequence of the opening in the palate. The mouth when presented for treatment had the appearance shown in Fig. 122.

A velum was made which restored the uvula in the lower flap, and in upper flap reproduced the septum of the interior nares where it was absent, also the posterior nares with its two openings.

FIG. 122.

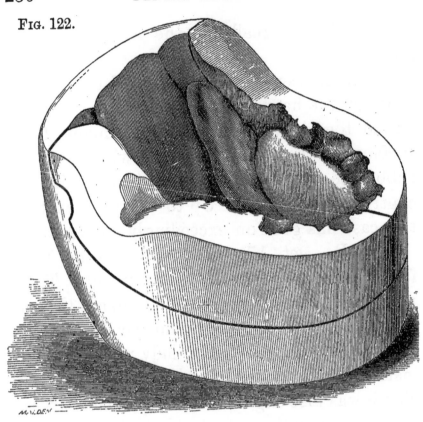

FIG. 123.

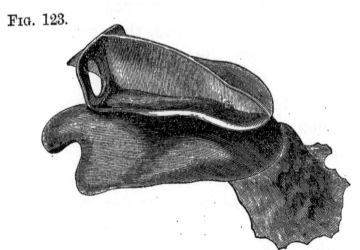

The artificial velum and front piece attached by means of the
platina pin.

By these means the mouth, nose, and upper part of the pharynx were restored to their natural condition, and much satisfaction was afforded by the improvement in a very short

FIG. 124.

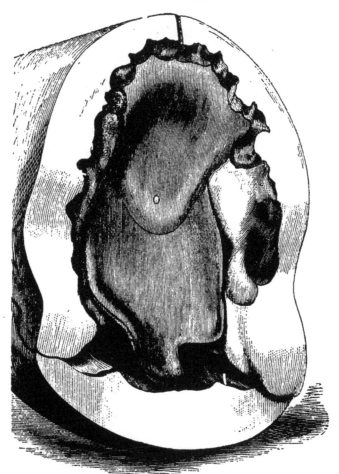

The mouth, as artificially restored.

time, not only in the facility with which the patient could make herself understood, but also

in the tone of the voice, which was unques-
tionably owing to the alterations that had been
produced in the form of the superior part of the
pharynx.

D. W—, æt. 38.—Consulted me in June,
1869, in reference to a cleft in his mouth, extending through the hard and soft palate and
alveolar ridge; there was an overlap on one
side of the cleft only, the opposite margin
articulating with the vomer.

An instrument was made of the form shown
in Figs. 125 and 126. The drawings illustrate

FIG. 125.

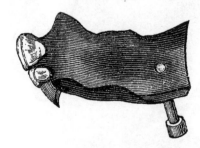

FIG. 126.

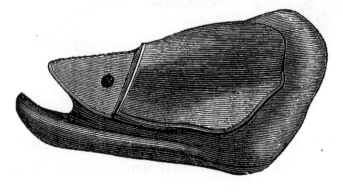

the manner in which the two parts are united, so as to present a smooth surface in the palate —a point of very great importance, where, under the most favorable circumstances, there is great difficulty in articulating with clearness. In this case it will be seen, as .in the previous ones, the artificial velum is held up by the overlap, and not by any attachments round the teeth.

W. H—, æt. 68.—Cleft of hard and soft palate, the harelip having been treated early in life; both the upper and lower jaws were without teeth. The appearance of the upper jaw, with the cleft, is shown in Fig. 127. A lower set of artificial teeth was being worn at the time; and I was desired to close the cleft without producing any irritation in the nasal cavity. I therefore made an ordinary full upper set of teeth, and continued backwards from its posterior border an artificial velum of elastic rubber, simply covering the cleft without any overlap. The form was, however, so simple that I think it unnecessary to give a drawing of it. The upper piece was connected with the lower by means of spiral springs, and fulfilled the special object it was made for in a most satisfactory manner, the patient having recovered and remained well ever since.

FIG. 127.

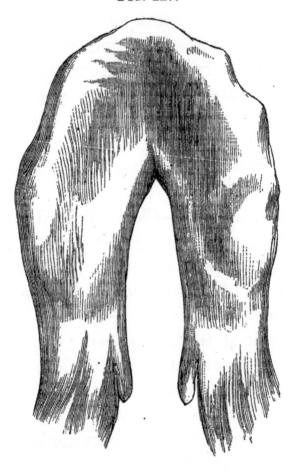

Miss W—, æt 19.—Brought to me March, 1869, suffering from thickness of speech, and inability to give the letters M, N, B, P, &c., with clearness. The young lady had suffered from enlarged tonsils, and had improved in utterance and general health since they had been removed, but her friends had still great difficulty in understanding her when reading;

and when she suffered from cold, even during ordinary conversation, she found a difficulty in making herself understood. The roof of the mouth was very high, and the dental arch much contracted. It was not thought desirable that anything should be done to remedy the contraction of the circle of the teeth, but an artificial palate was made to reduce the roof of the mouth to its normal depth.

Fig. 128 shows in section the peculiarity in

FIG. 128.

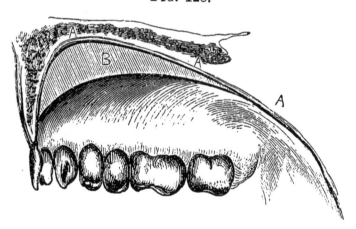

the shape of the palate (A, A), and at the same time shows the manner in which it was restored by means of a hard rubber plate (B). Within three weeks the speech was much clearer, and the voice more agreeable in sound. At the present time, while the palate is worn, both voice and speech are almost perfect.

16

The construction of an instrument for this purpose is so simple that it is not necessary to say more than that the impression having been taken in plaster of Paris, the palate was restored with wax to the proper shape, and the model put in the flask and packed with rubber in the usual way. After vulcanizing, it was finished off very carefully, so as to give a thin edge to the borders, and not offer any obstruction to the action of the tongue. The portion coming in contact with the palate should be left unpolished, and, in fact, untouched, beyond washing off the plaster, in order that better suction may be obtained when it is fitted in the mouth.

Miss M. R—, æt. 12.—Brought to me June, 1869, with elongated palate and projecting incisor teeth. The history of the case showed most unmistakeably that the deformity arose from sucking the thumb during infancy and childhood; and the evidence of the mother—a lady of great intelligence—confirmed this view. She said, when she had severe pain herself, she was in the habit of sucking her thumb as a diversion from the suffering, and her three female children had got into a similar custom, without any occasion but that of imitation. The deformity was not hereditary, as both father and mother had well-formed dental arches, and rather flat than deep palates. I extracted the first bicuspid on each side of the upper jaw, and made a vulcanite plate capping the side teeth, and having a broad band of elastic rubber, vulcanized with it, and passing in front of the incisors and canines, these teeth having been first reduced in the front, in order that sufficient pressure might be brought to bear upon them. In two months the teeth were brought into a fair position, considering the severity of the case. The projection of the lip was entirely reduced, but the teeth had an appearance—that is not uncommon in these cases—of being too long. The child will probably, however, grow out of this in a few years, as the whole of the face increases in size.

Syphilitic perforations of the palate are generally in the median line, though not always, and are more frequently of an oval than round shape, having their long diameter from back to front. There is not simply a loss of substance clearly defined, but the hole is bevelled off at the expense of its palatine surface, thus giving it a funnel-shaped appearance. This condition is usually found in perforations of the anterior third of the hard palate. I have never seen anything like it in the more posterior positions, or in the soft palate. Where there is simply a hole through the soft palate, there is generally, and I have as a rule found, considerable induration and thickening of the parts.

When the ulceration has gone on to such an extent as to produce cleft of the palate, there are often also present strong cicatrices, drawing the cleft widely apart, sometimes in a symmetrical position, and occasionally to one side of the pharynx. In some cases I have seen the uvula adherent to the back of the pharynx, or drawn down to one side, and almost touching the pillars of the fauces; while in others it has been strained forwards and downwards and attached by strong bands of flesh to the sides of the base of the tongue. I have seen, but only rarely, cleft of the palate with but small loss of substance, so that the two halves hung down into the pharynx, and occasionally caused great irritation from coming into contact with the epiglottis, and occasionally entire loss of the soft palate. In the condition of palate I am now describing examination with the rhinoscope will generally show considerable, if not entire destruction, of the opening of the posterior nares, or, speaking more correctly, the partition of the naso-pharyngeal cavities. The septum will be found much reduced in depth, and the whole of the upper portion of the space furnishing many points of resemblance to congenital cleft-palate.

Above the margin of the cleft, and springing out from the sides of the pharynx, there are frequently seen large nodulated masses of flesh; having sometimes the appearance of polypi, and not unlikely to be mistaken for them. They are, however, simply syphilitic outgrowths, and, once carefully examined, easily recognised again by their hardness to the touch and general consistency.

Judging from the cases I have treated, perforation of the soft palate is more frequent than that of the hard, while cleft of both hard and soft is more frequent than either.

It is well to mention that, occasionally, after the palate has been restored to such a state as to enable the patient to speak distinctly as to articulation, still the voice has an exceedingly disagreeable sound. On examining the throat with the laryngoscope, it will probably be found that this arises from some syphilitic affection of the larynx, such as ulceration of the epiglottis or of one or both of the vocal cords, or adhesion of the two vocal cords, to each other in a portion of their free borders, thus impeding vocalization; or there may be, as Dr Morell-

Mackenzie has pointed out, paralysis of some of the muscles of the larynx, produced by pressure of cicatrices or injury to a nerve-filament. This I mention to account for want of complete success in some of these cases. Another condition that affects the voice is the deafness often present in these cases, from ulceration or blocking up with growths of the opening of the Eustachian tubes. Some of the instances show that it is utterly impossible to reproduce the conditions necessary for perfect voice and speech, the difficulties being even greater than in congenital cleft palate.

Taking the impression.—It occasionally happens that the opening of the mouth is very much contracted, either from the effect of old cicatrices or gunshot wounds. This contraction may render it impossible to get a complete impression of the palate out of the mouth at one time.

To overcome this difficulty I have had a tray made of the form shown in Fig. 129, still in the shape of a spoon, but in two pieces, the handle of each overlapping the other; so that when the handles are brought into proper contact you may be quite sure that the two halves inside the mouth are in proper relative position to each other also.

The use of this sort of impression plate requires a little patience and skill to manage nicely, but there is no more difficulty than any one with ordinary tact will be able to overcome.

It may be used either with or without gutta percha on its surface. If gutta percha be used,

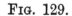

FIG. 129.

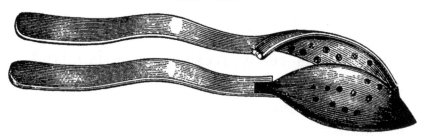

care must be taken to roughen it, in order to give attachment to the plaster of Paris. If this be neglected, the liability is incurred of leaving the plaster in the mouth, and bringing the tray away alone.

The one half of the tray is thus covered with a sufficient quantity of plaster, according to the case under treatment, and placed carefully on one side of the mouth, in such a position as to get a fair half of the impression, the right half of the spoon, of course, being used for the right side of the mouth. When the plaster is well set, it is carefully removed from the mouth, and the side which, with its fellow, is to form the median line of contact, pared down quite smooth, and flush with the edge of the spoon. The second half of the tray is then placed in its proper position with its fellow, to see that no overhanging portion of plaster is present before putting them into the mouth.

All the surface of the half impression already obtained is then soaped thoroughly with brown Windsor soap, by means of a camel's hair brush moistened either with water or sweet oil. When this is ready, fresh plaster is mixed in the manner hereafter described, and the impression already obtained is then placed again in the mouth in the exact position it first occupied, and held firmly in place by an assistant, or the patient, if he has sufficient intelligence and nerve to be trusted. The second half is now covered with a sufficient quantity of plaster, and introduced into the mouth, so as to obtain an impression of the parts left exposed, after the first impression is in position. The guide, as to the situation of the moist plaster in the mouth, is given to the operator by means of the perfect apposition of the two handles, which should have all their edges flush with each other.

At the time of placing the second impression in the mouth, the head should be thrown forwards, and to one side, that is, to the right, supposing the impression has been obtained of the right side first. This will have the effect of bringing plenty of plaster into the central portion of the palate, and so produce a more accurate impression than if the head is kept perfectly straight.

When the plaster in the basin indicates that the impression is sufficiently hard to bear removal, the first half—not the last—must be detached from its fellow in the mouth. A firm, quick pressure downwards will do this; a sufficient amount of space will then be found to remain inside the mouth to admit of its removal without suffering injury from dragging against the teeth.

By the time the first half is fairly removed, the second half will be sufficiently increased in strength to bear taking away without any chance of damage. We now have the two halves of the impression out of the mouth; and if the directions I have just given have been carefully carried out, there should be no difficulty in articulating them with each other. They will be best kept in contact by means of binding wire tied round the handles, and the two articulating surfaces being coated with liquid silex.

The perfect impression may then be cast in the usual way, or modified according to the nature of the case.

Treatment.—There is one rule that I think should be strictly adhered to in all cases of perforation of the hard and soft palate, and in most cases of cleft of the hard and soft palate when it arises from ulceration, and that is, never to introduce anything into the cavity of the perforation or cleft for permanent use. The tendency of the parts is to grow together, and thus gradually obliterate the opening.

Anything rising above the lower margin has the effect of checking this, and ultimately increasing rather than reducing the size of the space. In all these cases it is most essential that nothing shall be done to produce irritation and set up ulceration again.

The surface of the rubber coming next to the part of the palate where there is an opening must be highly polished, so that no chafing may take place. It should be flat rather than convex, so as to offer every inducement to the parts to come together.

The earlier these cases are treated the better they succeed, both as to the general health and the object we have specially in view, of remedying the defect in the palate. The plate preserves the parts from the irritation of foreign bodies, and the membranes are in such a condition as to grow more rapidly than under ordinary circumstances they would do.

I think it safest, and therefore best, to use black rubber for the plates, in order to avoid any possibility of injurious effects arising from the colouring matter used in the manufacture of the ordinary red dental rubber. For cleft and perforations of the velum it is generally necessary to use elastic rubber, but wherever it is possible to use hard rubber it is more efficient, if it be desired to reduce the size of an opening.

On this account, I sometimes use hard rubber for the front of the palate ; then a hinge formed of elastic rubber, and then hard rubber again beyond. This involves a little trouble in making, but the satisfactory results amply repay for the extra labour.

All the cases are held in position by the perfect fit of the plates to the mouth and teeth. I do not use bands or metallic collars round the teeth, and I never depend for the support of the pieces on any overlap to be obtained on the upper borders of the palate ; in syphilis I think this is too great a risk to run. When the perforation is in the hard palate, the plate may be made of such a shape as to cover it without unnecessarily encroaching on the roof of the mouth; when the opening is in the soft palate, the rubber should extend about $\frac{1}{8}$ to $\frac{1}{4}$ in. beyond the sides and back of the cavity. A case of this nature is shown in Fig. 130.

FIG. 130.

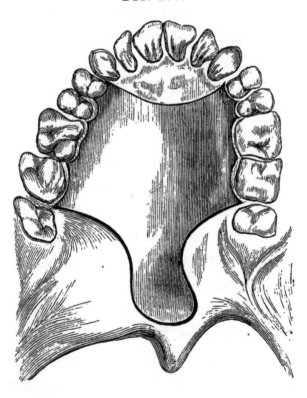

When there is a cleft, with the remains of the velum on each side attached to, and continuous with, the pharynx, it is neither possible nor desirable to close the cleft. The object here should be to stimulate the rigid margins and cicatrices into muscular action, in order that the naso-pharyngeal cavities may be separated at will. The hard rubber—for that is generally the best in the first instance, though elastic rubber may be used subsequently—should be fitted to within $\frac{1}{16}$ in. round the sides, and $\frac{1}{8}$ to $\frac{1}{4}$ in. at the portion coming in front of the posterior wall of the pharynx. The object of the difference in the dimensions of these spaces is that we desire to utilise and increase the lateral contractile power, while we leave the muscles at the back of the pharynx in their normal condition, simply letting them touch the border of the obturator without impinging.

It must be borne in mind that it is most essential for the health of the patient that the mucus of the nose should not be allowed to accumulate to an unnatural degree, by the complete closure of the space between the posterior nares and mouth; added to which, it is necessary to avoid the chance of the artificial palate being thrown out of position by the tilting up of the margin coming in contact with the pharynx.

In two cases, where there were no teeth in the upper jaw, the obturator was held in position by means of spiral springs attached to a lower piece.

The models must be taken in plaster of Paris, but as there are occasionally perforations too large to be covered with gold-beater's skin (to prevent the plaster entering), there is a risk of some considerable portion of it remaining in the opening when the impression is removed. I have, therefore, had constructed an instrument fashioned like a lithotrite, which, by being introduced into the opening, enables the operator to crush the plaster, and then remove it with a pair of tweezers, and afterwards wash away the fragments with a syringe and warm water.

This instrument is shown in Fig. 131.*

FIG. 131.

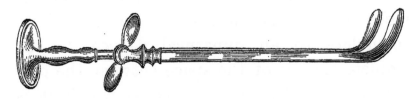

Making the Palate Plates.—For all practical purposes, hard and elastic rubber may be vulcanized together, providing the temperature is sufficiently high to thoroughly cook the hard rubber.

* Made by Meyer and Metzler, Great Portland Street.

The elastic rubber does not suffer from this increased temperature in elasticity, but in power of resisting the acids of the mouth. Still, it is sometimes desirable to put up with this disadvantage on account of the other benefits to be derived from the practice. It is necessary when this is done to vulcanize on metallic moulds, either fitted in a flask or held together by a clamp.

The model having been cast in plaster, is moulded in sand and cast carefully in type-metal. All that portion of the palate which has been recently the seat of ulceration is well polished, so as to bring it up to a high metallic surface.

Then, instead of mounting up the form of the plate in wax, as you would do on a plaster model, use modelling clay tolerably dry, that is, as dry as it can be worked conveniently. When it is nicely finished up, and has the form the artificial palate is to have in rubber, whether hard or soft, it is placed by the fire and gradually dried and made warm on the type-metal model; it is afterwards placed in a casting-ring, with sand round it—in the same way that we proceed for making the lead counterpart for plate work—and type-metal poured in. This saves the time and trouble of making a plaster model first, and also insures a more accurate fit of the two castings.

All the surface of this last casting is thoroughly polished, so as to give a smooth surface to the rubber. The rubber is afterwards packed in according to the position that you desire the hard and elastic portions of it to occupy. It is then fixed in a clamp and vulcanized.

Cases.—Sophia S—, æt. 32.—Applied at the Hospital for Diseases of the Throat for treatment of severe ulceration and loss of parts at the back of the mouth. Nearly the whole of the velum palati had disappeared, the anterior and posterior pillars of the fauces were likewise destroyed, so that the roof of the mouth presented the appearance of continuance backwards to the posterior wall of the pharynx, as shown in Fig. 132.

In the position that would be occupied by the uvula and central portion of the soft palate, when elevated for dividing the mouth from the nose, there was a large opening of an oval form, about one and a quarter of an inch in extent one way, and three quarters of an inch from side to side. In swallowing, there was not the slightest movement at the back of the mouth, except in the tongue, which was the only member that could contribute any assistance to

FIG. 132.

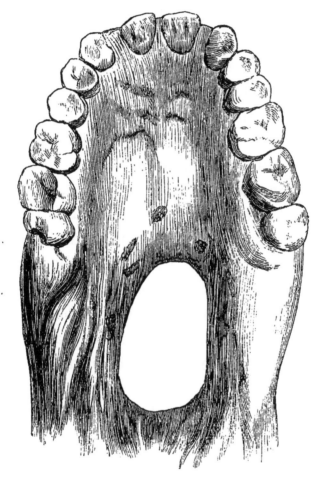

Showing cicatrices and old syphilitic scars in front of fissure.

the process of conveying the food to the opening into the œsophagus. The back of the
mouth was in this way kept in a very irritable
condition by the continual lodgment of food in
the cleft. From the state of the palate, speech
was scarcely intelligible, and the life of the

17

poor woman was in every way a matter of considerable discomfort. Owing also to the great induration of the parts on each side, where the indications of the anterior pillars of the fauces were apparent, I concluded that no power could be obtained to work an elastic velum with any service or comfort, while at the same time there was the consideration to be borne in mind that the disease was still going on, and it was desirable rather to protect the parts from the irritation resulting from food, &c., than to increase the trouble by having an artificial velum, that must necessarily produce some chafing, the mucous membrane being so exceedingly sensitive. A simple hard rubber obturator was therefore made, partially closing the aperture, and having the inner surface highly polished. This has been very satisfactory in its results.

William T—, engineer, æt. 37.—In this case the upper maxillary bone was destroyed on the left side from the central tooth to the second molar tooth, following the line of the intermaxillary suture, and the connection of the palate-bone with the upper maxilla. The septum of the nose was quite perfect, articulating with the maxillary bone of the opposite side. The turbinated bones of the left side, with the walls of the antrum, were entirely destroyed up to the floor of the orbit, leaving a gap for restoration by artificial means of considerable extent. The voice was very imperfect, mastication and swallowing very difficult.

FIG. 133.

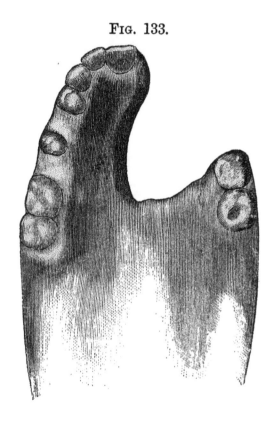

The instrument that was constructed to remedy these defects is shown complete, ready for wear, in Fig. 134.

The means that were adopted were not only satisfactory, but immediate in their result—

FIG. 134.

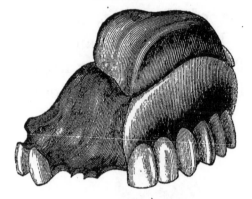

The parts connected ready for wear.

FIG. 135.

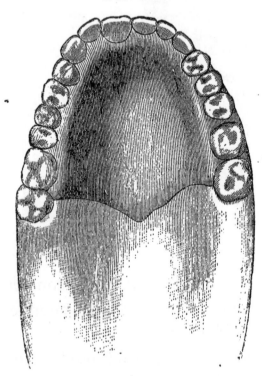

The mouth as artificially restored.

speech was restored at once to its normal tone and distinctness. Gargling the throat and mouth (before impossible) were now accomplished with ease, while by the restoration of the teeth to their natural state the patient's appearance was very much improved. The appearance of the mouth after treatment is shown in Fig. 135.

The deformities arising from **phagedænic ulceration** must be treated on precisely the same principle as those arising from syphilitic ulceration; it is not therefore necessary to enter into these separately.

The deformities of the mouth arising from **mechanical injury** assume the most various conditions, consisting either of defect owing to loss of substance, or malformation dependent on the influence of cicatrices of wounds inflicted in the soft tissues. In the former instance we have simply to reproduce the lost parts as nearly like nature as possible, but in the latter it may be necessary to construct an apparatus or appliance in such a way as to counteract and at last overcome the disfigurement arising from the steady contraction of the flesh.

Each case must be treated according to its special features and peculiarities. No precise instruction can be of any use. Certain general

rules of action may, however, be of service.   On
every occasion when these deformities come
under treatment, make it a first, and hold it the
most important step to obtain a perfect model,
and always with plaster of Paris.   For taking
the impression, if ordinary trays are not available make especial ones ; if there is not room to
place the tray in position with the plaster in it,
then contrive an opening in an accessible portion
of the impression cup, and after it is in the mouth
in its proper position fill up the intervening
space between the plate and the part to be
modelled, with very thin plaster of Paris in-
jected by means of a large-mouthed syringe ;
in this way impressions very accurate in character may be obtained of apparently the most
awkward and inaccessible parts of the mouth.

In reproducing the defective parts use soft
or elastic rubber to supply soft parts, and hard
rubber to fill up the gap or deficiency in hard
tissue ; this is a rule that nearly always holds
good.   Where you have no diseased condition
present always obtain a given and, if possible,
perfect result by the most simple method you
can adopt.   Let ingenuity be applied to sim-
plifying an apparatus rather than to making
it curious in character and complicated in construction.   Rest assured that your patient will be

best pleased with that appliance which answers most perfectly and gives the least trouble rather than with one that shows contriving skill on the part of the operator, but from its structure is likely to get easily out of repair and always be a source of anxiety for its safety.

APPENDIX

RECEIPTS FOR MAKING GOLD PLATE OF THE VARIOUS QUALITIES MOST IN USE FOR THE MOUNTING OF ARTIFICIAL DENTURES.*

GOLD PLATE EIGHTEEN CARATS FINE.

Formula, No. 1.

18 dwts. pure gold,
4 dwts. fine copper,
2 dwts. fine silver.

Formula, No. 2.

20 dwts. gold coin,
2 dwts. fine copper,
2 dwts. fine silver.

GOLD PLATE NINETEEN CARATS FINE.

Formula, No. 3.

19 dwts. pure gold,
3 dwts. copper,
2 dwts. silver.

Formula, No. 4.

20 dwts. gold coin,
25 grains of copper,
40 + grs. of silver.

* Richardson and Harris, op. cit.

GOLD PLATE TWENTY CARATS FINE.

Formula, No. 5.
20 dwts. pure gold,
2 dwts. copper,
2 dwts. silver.

Formula, No. 6.
20 dwts. gold coin,
18 grs. copper,
20 + grs. silver.

GOLD PLATE TWENTY-ONE CARATS FINE.

Formula, No. 7.
20 dwts. pure gold,
2 dwts. copper,
1 dwt. silver.

Formula, No. 8.
20 dwts. gold coin,
13 + grs. silver.

Formula, No. 9.
20 dwts. gold coin,
6 grs. copper,
$7\frac{5}{7}$ grs. platinum.

GOLD PLATES TWENTY-TWO CARATS FINE.

Formula, No. 10.
22 dwts. pure gold,
1 dwt. fine copper,
18 grs. silver,
6 grs. platinum.

SOLDERS FOR GOLD WORK.

The following formula may be used in connection with eighteen or twenty carat gold plate, and is sixteen carats fine.

6 dwts. pure gold,
2 dwts. roset copper,
1 dwt. fine silver.

Formula No. 1 of the following recipes is a fraction over fifteen carats fine; and No. 2 furnishes a solder eighteen carats fine.

Formula No. 1.
6 dwts. gold coin,
30 grs. silver,
20 grs. copper, .
10 grs. brass.

Formula No. 2.
Gold coin, 30 parts,
Silver   4   ,,
Copper   1   ,,
Brass   1   ;

SILVER SOLDER.

Formula No. 1.
Silver   66 parts,
Copper 30   ,,
Zinc   10   ,,

Formula, No 2.
Silver   6 parts,
Copper 2   ,,
Brass 1   ,,

BRASS SOLDER.

Brass solder consists of two parts of brass and one of zinc, to which a little tin is occasionally added.

SOFT SOLDER.

Soft solder is an alloy composed of lead and tin in the proportion of two parts of the former with one of the latter.

ROSE'S FUSIBLE METAL.

The alloy known as Rose's *fusible metal* is composed of 2 parts of bismuth, 1 of lead, and 1 of tin, and melts at about 200°. A still more fusible alloy is composed of lead 3 parts, tin 2 parts, and bismuth 5 parts, which fuses at 197°.

RABBITT'S METAL.

Melt 4 lbs. of copper; add by degrees 12 lbs. of tin and 8 lbs. of antimony. Then add 12 lbs. more tin, first by adding 4 lbs., bring the whole to a red heat and then add the rest of the tin.

GERMAN SILVER.

Genuine *German silver* is composed of copper 40·4; nickel 31·6; zinc 25·4; iron 2·6; but the proportions of the metals of this alloy differ according to the various uses to which this compound is applied.

TYPE METAL.

Lead, alloyed with antimony in the proportion of from $\frac{1}{4}$ to $\frac{1}{8}$ of the latter, with the addition sometimes of very small portions of copper, tin, and bismuth, forms different grades of *type metal,* which is harder than lead, and very brittle, and is sometimes used for dies; and sometimes, though very rarely, for counter-dies. When used as a counter to a zinc die, it is improved for the purpose by adding to it an equal quantity of lead; it may also be used in the form of a die in connection with a lead counter after rough stamping with zinc.

METHOD OF REDUCING GOLD TO A LOWER OR HIGHER STANDARD OF FINENESS AND OF DETERMINING THE CARAT OF ANY GIVEN ALLOY.

The following practical remarks on the method are copied from an article on "Alloying Gold,"* by Professor G. Watt.

" 1. *To ascertain the carat of any given alloy.*— The proportion may be expressed as follows :

" As the weight of the alloyed mass is to the weight of gold it contains, so is 24 to the standard sought. Take for example, Harris' No. 3 gold solder :

Pure gold	6	parts,
„ silver	2	„
„ copper	1	„
Total . . .	9	

* 'Dental Register of the West,' vol. x, p. 396.

" The proportion would be expressed thus,—

$$9 : 6 :: 24 : 16.$$

" From this any one can deduce the following

" RULE.—Multiply 24 by the weight of gold in the alloyed mass, and divide the product by the weight of the mass; the quotient is the carat sought.

" In the above example, 24 multiplied by 6, the quantity of gold, gives 144, which, divided by 9, the weight of the whole mass, gives 16. Hence, an alloy prepared as above, is 16 carats fine.

" As another example, under the same rule, take Harris' No. 1 solder.

22 carat gold, 48 parts,
silver, 16   „
copper, 12   „
—
Total . . . 76

" Now, as the gold used is but 22 carats fine, one twelfth of it is alloy. The one twelfth of 48 is 4, which subtracted from 48 leaves 44. The statement then is :

$$76 : 44 :: 241 : 3\cdot9.$$

" This solder, therefore, falls a fraction below 14 carats.

" 2. *To reduce gold to a required carat.*— The proportion may be expressed as follows :

" As the required carat is to 24, so is the weight of the gold used to the weight of the alloyed mass when reduced. The weight of gold subtracted from this, gives the quantity of alloy to be added.

" For example, reduce 6 ounces of pure gold to 16 carats.

" The statement is expressed thus :

$$16 : 24 :: 6 : 9.$$

" Six subtracted from 9 leaves 3, which is the quantity of alloy to be added. From this is deducted the following

" RULE.—Multiply 24 by the weight of pure gold used, and divide the product by the required carat. The quotient is the weight of the mass when reduced, from which subtract the weight of the gold used, and the remainder is the weight of alloy to be added.

" As another example under the same rule, reduce 1 pennyweight of 22 carat gold to 18 carats.

" As the gold is only 22 carats fine, one twelfth of it is already alloy. The one pennyweight, therefore, contains but twenty-two grains of pure gold. The statement is, therefore, thus expressed :

$$18 : 24 :: 22 : 29\tfrac{1}{3}.$$

" Twenty-two subtracted from $29\tfrac{1}{3}$ leaves $7\tfrac{1}{3}$.

Therefore, each pennyweight of 22 carat gold requires $7\frac{1}{3}$ grains of alloy to reduce it to 18 carats.

"3. *To reduce gold from a lower to a higher carat.*—This may be done by adding pure gold, or a gold alloy finer than that required. The principle of the rule may be set forth in the following general expression:

"As the alloy in the required carat is to the alloy in the given carat, so is the weight of the alloyed gold used to the weight of the reduced alloy required. The principle may be practically applied by the following

"RULE.—Multiply the weight of the alloyed gold used by the number representing the proportion of alloy in the given carat, and divide the product by that representing the proportion of alloy in the required carat; the quotient is the weight of the mass when reduced to the required carat by adding fine gold.

"To illustrate this, take the following example:

"Reduce 1 pennyweight of 16 carat gold to 18 carats.

"The numbers representing the proportions of alloy in this example are found by respectively subtracting 18 and 16 from 24. The statement is, therefore:

$$6 : 8 :: 1 : 1\tfrac{1}{3},$$

from which it follows that to reduce one penny-weight of 16 carat gold to 18 carats, there must be one third of a pennyweight of pure gold added to it.

"But, suppose that, instead of pure gold, we wish to effect the change by adding 22 carat gold. The numbers, then, respectively representing the proportions of the alloy would be found by subtracting, in the above example, 16 and 18 from 22, and the statement would be

$$4 : 6 :: 1 : 1\tfrac{1}{2}.$$

"It follows, then, that to each pennyweight of 16 carat gold, a half pennyweight of 22 carat gold must be added to bring it to 18 carats.

"By the above rules we think the student will be able, in all cases, to calculate the fineness or quality of his gold, and to effect any reduction, whether ascending or descending, which he may desire."

DR HUNTER'S METHOD OF SUPPORTING PARTIAL DENTURES IN THE MOUTH BY MEANS OF CYLINDERS OF WOOD ATTACHED TO TUBED PLATES.

Dr Hunter remarks:—"The advantages in many cases must be apparent to the thinking dentist, but, perhaps, it might not be amiss to enumerate a few.

" The fixture is held in place with greater firmness than by means of clasps.

" In some instances where I have used clasps, I have also used the tube in combination, to give stability for masticating purposes.

" The injury to the natural teeth must be much less, owing to the smaller amount of surface in contact.

" If decay should take place, it would require but an ordinary filling to restore the tooth.

" It prevents that peculiarly disagreeable sensation experienced, particularly in fruit season, upon removing and replacing artificial teeth.

" After having tested it for more than a year, I am satisfied that it greatly lessens the chances of decay in those cases where it can be applied, and I have removed the clasps in some old cases with great satisfaction to my patients."

TABLE SHOWING THE NAMES, COLOURS, AND DEGREES
OF HEAT REQUIRED FOR VULCANIZING THE RUB-
BERS THAT ARE MOST USED AT THE PRESENT
TIME

C. Ash and Sons' Rubbers.

Names.	Colours.	Time.		Degrees Fahr.	Degrees Cent.	Degrees Réamur.
		h.	m.			
1x	Deep pink ...	⎫				
1x, soft	„ „ ...	⎬ 1	15	310	154	124
No. 1	Pale „ ...					
No. 2	Light „ ...	⎭				
G	Bright red ...	2	0	315	157	126
Ord. 12/-	Deep red	2	0	315	157	126
Ord. 10/-	Brown	2	0	315	157	126
Black	...	2	0	315	157	126
S. P.	Strong pink..	1	45	315	157	126
White...	...	1	15	315	157	126
Red	...	1	15	315	157	126
Orange	...	1	15	315	157	126
Brown........	...	1	15	315	157	126
Soft	Red	1	15	310	154	124
W.	Dark brown...	1	15	310	154	124
Whalebone .	Light brown	0	50	320	160	127
		⎧ 2	0	240	115	92
Vela	Brown	⎨ 2	· 0	260	126	101
		⎩ 2	0	270	132	106
A/E........ . ..	Dark red	1	15	310	154	124
American Whalebone Rubber	Deep red ...	0	55	320	160	127

In the course of some experiments that I
carried out four years ago with various rubbers
I found that nearly all of them could be rendered elastic, like the vela rubber, by raising
the heat gradually to the point of vulcanization

and then at once cooling down. To those who may at any time find it difficult to obtain the elastic rubber required for an artificial velum this fact may be of service.

TO OBTAIN SUCTION

After a perfect model has been taken and an artificial piece accurately fitted, the operator is often much perplexed to find that the plate will not hold up. In many cases this arises from nervousness on the part of the patient, causing the secretion of mucus to be arrested, and thus altering the condition of the surface of the mouth sufficiently to prevent suction being obtainable. The best remedy is to paint over the palate and adjacent gums with a solution of carbolic acid and glycerine (1 in 12) ; this will stimulate the action of the mucous follicles, and in a short time perfect adhesion of the plate to the palate will take place.

REPAIRING VULCANITE

Vulcanite cases may sometimes be successfully repaired and have teeth added to them by means of soft solder applied with a small soldering iron. The dovetails are cut in the usual way, and the soft solder run in, the piece being supported by a plaster mould made warm, but not hot enough to injure the rubber.

TO RESTORE VULCANITE CASES TO THEIR FIRST FORM

Vulcanite plates are sometimes made warm by means of hot oil or the spirit lamp, so that they may be altered in shape. Occasionally this is done with very unsatisfactory results, and it becomes desirable to restore the piece to its first form. This may be done by immersing the plate for a few minutes in boiling water.

SPIRAL SPRINGS

I have intentionally omitted any notice of the application of spiral springs in the body of this work, as I believe they no longer hold a prominent place in modern dentistry, and only proper care is required in the adjustment of full upper dentures to enable the operator to do without springs altogether.

There are, however, sometimes cases where the prejudices of a patient will compel you to fix spiral springs, or else see your work thrown aside as useless. Until our patients are better educated in regard to these matters, spiral springs will therefore occasionally be called into use. They are attached to the upper and lower set by means of swivels.

The swivel consists of a pin made of platinum or gold passing through the " eye;" to this latter is joined the shank, to which the spring itself is attached ; the swivel in its complete form may be connected to a vulcanite base by the pin passing through the vulcanite and being riveted on the lingual surface, or for a gold case it may be mounted on a small plate, and attached by soldering to the side of the denture.

Supposing the jaws to be normally developed, the best position for the swivels is between the second bicuspid and first molar in either jaw; the swivels in the lower jaw will then be somewhat in advance of the upper jaw when the teeth are closed, but will fall in the same perpendicular line when the lower jaw is depressed. If when the mouth is closed the swivels are opposite to each other, that is, fall in the same line, when the mouth is opened the upper swivels will occupy a position in advance of the lower ones, and the springs, having thus lost their proper balance, will occasionally project the teeth out of the mouth, often partially and sometimes altogether.

The manufacture of spiral springs has been already mentioned in the section on gold. The various forms of swivels, and their adjustment with the springs to a full set of teeth, are shown in the accompanying woodcuts.

FIG. 136.

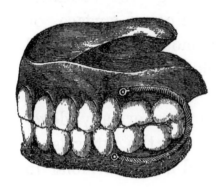

FIG. 137.

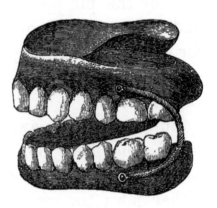

FIG. 138.

FIG. 139.

FIG. 140.

TO PREVENT ABRASION OF THE CHEEK FROM SPIRAL SPRINGS

When it is necessary to use spiral springs for the first time, much discomfort is often endured by the patient on account of the chafing produced by them. This may be, in a great measure, prevented or relieved by one or other of the following plans :—Either make a solution in chloroform of pink rubber and paint over the surface of the springs before putting them on the set of teeth, or else obtain some of the very fine and thin elastic rubber tubing which is now made; and, having first passed a brooch up the centre of the spring to prevent crippling, draw this tubing over, so that the whole of it is covered except those portions that play against the teeth. In this way these necessary evils may be made tolerable to sensitive mouths by protecting the mucous membrane from their metallic feeling and irritation.

INDEX

PRINTED BY J. E. ADLARD, BARTHOLOMEW CLOSE, LONDON, E.C.